Science and Clinical Practice of Dental Caries

Science and Clinical Practice of Dental Caries

Edited by **Kaley Ann**

New Jersey

Published by Foster Academics,
61 Van Reypen Street,
Jersey City, NJ 07306, USA
www.fosteracademics.com

Science and Clinical Practice of Dental Caries
Edited by Kaley Ann

International Standard Book Number: 978-1-63242-360-3 (Hardback)

Printed in the United States of America.

Contents

Preface

This book discusses latest developments regarding the etiology, pathogenesis, diagnosis and treatment of caries. With such advancements, it will soon become possible to completely defeat dental caries. It comprises of basic information regarding dental caries and caries diagnosis. This book will be a valuable and rich source of information for students, practitioners, dentists and professionals engaged in this domain of medical science.

The book has been the outcome of endless efforts put in by authors and researchers on various issues and topics within the field. The book is a comprehensive collection of significant researches that are addressed in a variety of chapters. It will surely enhance the knowledge of the field among readers across the globe.

It is indeed an immense pleasure to thank our researchers and authors for their efforts to submit their piece of writing before the deadlines. Finally in the end, I would like to thank my family and colleagues who have been a great source of inspiration and support.

Editor

Part 1

The Caries

1

Caries Through Time:
An Anthropological Overview

Luis Pezo Lanfranco and Sabine Eggers

Laboratório de Antropologia Biológica, Depto. de Genética e Biologia Evolutiva,
Instituto de Biociências, Universidade de São Paulo,
Brazil

1. Introduction

Bioanthropological[1] researches carried out in the last few decades have given special emphasis to the study of the relation between disease, as well as social and environmental phenomena, enhancing the already strong connection between lifestyle and health conditions during history of humankind (Cohen & Armelagos, 1984; Katzenberg & Saunders, 2008; Larsen, 1997). Because infectious diseases result from the interaction between host and agent, modulated by ecological and cultural environments, the comparative study of the historic prevalence of diseases in past populations worldwide can provide important data about their related factors and etiology.

The study of dental diseases (such as caries) has been given special attention from Paleopathology[2]. The tooth, for its physical features tends to resist destruction and taphonomic conditions better than any other body tissue and therefore, is a valuable element for the study on individual's diet, and social and cultural factors related to it, from a population perspective.

Caries is one of the infectious diseases more easily observable in human remains retrieved from archaeological excavations. For their long time of development and non-lethal nature the lesions presented at the time of the death remain recognizable indefinitely, allowing to infer, along with other archaeological and ecological data, the types of food that a specific population consumed, the cooking technology they used, the relative frequency of consumption, and the way the food was shared among the group (Hillson, 2001 2008; Larsen, 1997; Rodríguez, 2003).

---

[1] Formerly called Physical Anthropology, Bioanthropology is a discipline that provides integrated information about the lifestyle of past populations and their associations with the environment through the study of human remains. The North American school denominates it Bioarchaeology (Buikstra & Beck, 2006; Larsen, 1997; Roberts & Manchester, 2005).

[2] In general, diseases, signs and determining factors have been studied by Bioanthropology under the label of Paleopathology (the study of diseases in past societies through ancient texts, art and human remains). The specific study of the oral diseases during ancient times is named Oral or Dental paleopathology (Campillo, 2001; Waldron, 2009).

Considering the available data, we know that the highest caries rates[3], their distribution and severity profiles observed nowadays are the result of a complex process of slow dietary changes, directly linked to the development of Western civilization. Consequently, the current caries patterns are not observed in past populations, on the opposite, they show a high variability along time and space that corresponds to a wide range of subsistence strategies, specific cultural regulations, and particular historical processes.

2. The antiquity of caries: Evidences of caries in hominines and early humans

Caries is a very old disease and it is not exclusive of the human species. Evidences of dental lesions compatible with caries have been observed in creatures as old as Paleozoic fishes (570-250 million years), Mesozoic herbivores dinosaurs (245-65 million years), pre-hominines of the Eocene (60-25 million years), and Miocenic (25-5 million years), Pliocenic (5-1.6 million years), and Pleistocenic animals (1.6-0.01 million years – Clement, 1958; Kear, 2001; Kemp, 2003; Sala et al., 2004). Caries has also been detected in bears and other wild animals (Pinto & Exteberria, 2001; Palamra et al., 1981), and it is common in domestic animals (Gorrel, 2006; Shklair, 1981; Wiggs & Lobprise, 1997).

In humans, caries is one of the most widely spread diseases and its presence takes place into our species origins. Paleodietary reconstructions have provided a high amount of data on the presence of caries in ancestral lineages. An approximal groove located in the cementum-enamel junction (CEJ) of bicuspids and molars has been noticed in several lineages of fossil hominines like Paranthropus robustus, Homo habilis, H. erectus, H. heidelbergensis and H. neanderthalensis (Bermúdez de Castro et al., 1997; Frayer, 1991; Milner & Larsen, 1991; Ungar et al., 2001). Although some scholars have reported that lesion as caries (Clement, 1956; Grine et al., 1990; Robinson, 1952), more recent analyses done in an specimen of Homo erectus from Olduvai Gorge (1.84 million years BP[4]) suggest that it could be an erosion produced by the habitual (possibly therapeutic) use of tooth-picks (Ungar et al., 2001).

Also, the paleopathological record of the ATE9-1 jaw (Homo sp. - Sima del Elefante site, Sierra de Atapuerca, Spain), considered the oldest hominine fossil of Western Europe (1.3 million years BP), shows numerous maxillary lesions such as hypercementosis, calculus deposits, periodontal disease, cystic lesions and an anomalous wear facet compatible with tooth picking but no caries (Martinón et al., 2011).

Several authors have suggested that the discovery of fire by Homo erectus-like species, around 800 thousand years ago, was a biologically significant step. Meanwhile cooked food replaced a

---

[3] Some prompts are used for the recording of caries experience. Caries prevalence, defined as the number of individuals in a population affected by caries in a specific time span. Caries frequency, defined as the number of teeth affected for caries divided by the total number of sockets observed (tooth/tooth socket) in a individual or population; and caries index as the Decay Missing Filling Index adapted to fragmentary samples (Duyar & Erdal, 2003; Lukacs, 1992; Medronho et al., 2009; Pezo, 2010; Saunders et al., 1997).

[4] The chronological dating methods use some conventional parameters. BP (before present) refers to a non- calibrated C14 date, calculated since 1950 as year zero. BC and AD (before Christ and Anno Domini respectively) refers to a calibrated C14 date (calculated from accurate historical or geological data) in calendar years since the year one of our era (Taylor, 1987).

diet entirely based on raw meat and vegetables, the patterns of chewing, digestion and nutrition changed accordingly. The process of cooking using fire turned the food safer, juicer, and easier to digest, promoting a higher intake of energy that, in evolutionary terms, had a sequence of favorable physiological effects. The easy digestion of cooked food would have favored the reduction of the digestive system, facilitating metabolic energy savings that were used to develop the brain (Aiello & Wheeler, 1995; Cartmill, 1993; Wrangham, 2009). Nevertheless, it is supposed that *H. erectus,* a hunter-gatherer, obtained approximately 50% of its calories from carbohydrates (Wrangham, 2009) and under the hypothesis of cooking (that obviously included meat and vegetables), caries should have been present much earlier in the fossil record. However, caries appears clearly much later. So, the data on oral does not support the idea of a cariogenic diet based on cooked vegetables from the earliest periods. Maybe, in the beginning, fire was employed only for cooking meat.

The unquestionable oldest evidence of caries comes from a fossil found in 1921 in Broken Hill, Northern Rhodesia (Zambia) during the exploration of a zinc mine. The specimen denominated Broken Hill 1, a *Homo rhodesiensis* cranium (African version of the *Homo heidelberguensis* 650,000-160,000 BP) shows extensive dental caries and coronal destruction. Except for five teeth, all the rest is affected by rampant caries and several crowns are almost completely destroyed. Caries seems to have its origin in the interdental spaces. Besides, Broken Hill man experienced alveolar recession and dental abscesses in many teeth (Fig. 1). Although lesions have been attributed to a diet rich in vegetables and/or poisoning by the existing metals in the region (Bartsiokas & Day, 1993), it seems that, given the interdental origin of the caries and the absence of tooth picks evidence, the Broken Hill 1 developed his lesions due to his ignorance in the use of tooth picks, which was known by other earlier hominines (Puech, 1978).

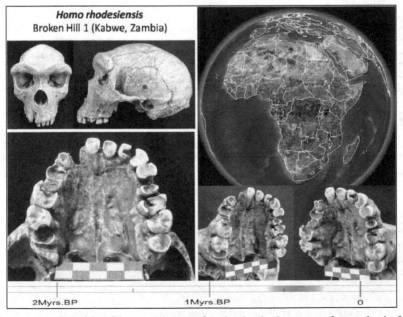

Fig. 1. **The unquestionable oldest evidence of caries in the human paleontological record.** Pictures of *H. rhodesiensis* skull cast. Map modified from Google Maps 2010.

In this sense, from the presence of caries in non-human primates one must consider that natural sources of carbohydrates can produce carious lesions. Caries have been reported in prime-age individuals of *Pongo pygmaeus* (4.1%), *Gorilla gorilla* (2.7%), *Hylobates* (0.9%) and *Pan troglodytes* (12.7% in juveniles versus 30.6% in older animals – Crovella & Ardito, 1994; Schultz, 1956). Thus, in modern apes, the disease exists despite them being mostly herbivorous with a raw diet based on only a few starchy tubers if any (Kilgore, 1995; Miles & Grigson, 1990).

The Neanderthals (230,000-30,000 BP) show a high prevalence of enamel hypoplasias, antemortem tooth loss, periodontal disease and abscesses but dental caries is very rare among them (Brennan, 1991; Brothwell, 1963; Grine et al., 1990; Ogilvie, 1989). Six cases (Table 1) of dental caries (0.48%) have been reported among the approximately 1250 known Neanderthal teeth (Lalueza et al., 1993; Lebel & Trinkaus, 2001; Tillier et al., 1995; Trinkaus et al., 2000; Walker et al., 2011). The presence of caries in Neanderthals suggests the existence of pathogenic dental plaque and dietary conditions compatible with the consumption of some cariogenic carbohydrates despite the hunter-gatherer lifestyle and cold climate existing during the Middle Paleolithic[5] (Trinkaus et al., 2000).

Specimen	Tooth	Description
Banyoles 1 France (Lalueza et al., 1993).	Mandibular M3	Two small pits with irregular shapes in occlusal fissures, penetration beyond the dento-enamel junctions.
Kebara 27 Israel (Tillier et al., 1995)	Maxillary I2	A cavity in the central pit of a strongly shoveled tooth, 2.6 mm diameter, extended through the dento-enamel junction.
Bau de l'Aubesier 5 France (Trinkaus et al., 2000)	Maxillary dm1	A mid-lingual pit lesion.
Bau de l'Aubesier 12 France (Lebel &Trinkaus, 2001)	Maxillary M1 or M2	A large hole across the disto-lingual corner of the cervical half of the roots, 7.2 mm high, 6.3 mm wide, 3.5 mm depth.
Sima de Palomas 25 Spain (Walker et al., 2011)	Mandibular dm1	An occlusal cavity, 1.2 mm diameter, extended through the exposed dentin.
Sima de Palomas 59 Spain (Walker et al., 2011)	MandibularM2	A small interproximal notch.

Table 1. Carious lesions among Neanderthals

---

[5] The Paleolithic or Antique Stone Age was the longest period of human prehistory (99% of it), ranging from 2.8 millions of years (in Africa) to 10,000 BP. The Paleolithic is divided in three periods: Lower Paleolithic (2.8 million years to 200,000 years: the epoch of the hominines and our first ancestors), Middle Paleolithic (the epoch of Neanderthals, from approximately 200,000 to 30,000 BP), and Upper Paleolithic (30,000 BP- 10,000 BP – the epoch of the earliest modern humans). The Neolithic or New Stone Age was defined considering the new way of life based on the production of food from domesticated species. It appears at different times and regions around the world during the Holocene (starts 10,000 BP). The phase of transition between the Paleolithic and Neolithic is known as Mesolithic (Carbonell, 2005).

Dental caries are present but still rare among early modern humans (European and Near Eastern *Homo sapiens*) during the Upper Paleolithic. Caries have been identified in Qafzeh 3 and Skhul 2 in Israel (Fryer, 1976; Boydstun et al., 1988), and only Cro-Magnon 4, Les Rois R50-4 and Les Rois R51-15 have been indentified with caries in Europe (Brennan, 1991; Trikanus et al., 2000). Caries are more widely found among more recent Eurasian foraging peoples, but caries frequencies remain below 10% (Brothwell, 1963; Caselitz, 1998).

3. Caries and lifestyle

3.1 Dietary changes and the raise of caries experience in past human societies

In fact, the history of dental caries is associated with the rise of civilization, and more recently with dietary changes that occurred since the Mercantilism and Industrial Revolution. Several archaeological and historical works have confirmed the relationship between high caries frequencies and prevalences and the increase of carbohydrates intake in human populations from the advent of agriculture[6] (Larsen, 1997; Saunders et al., 1997; Turner, 1979). Generally hunter-gatherers show low caries frequencies whereas peoples based on mixed economies, gardening, and farming, show increasingly higher caries rates (Hillson, 2001; Lukacs, 1992; Powell, 1985; Turner, 1979).

For instance, in the North American Southeast the number of carious teeth in farmers is three times the number of carious teeth in foragers of prior epochs (Powell, 1985). In several populations from Eastern Woodlands of North America the changes are also observed along the time, with frequencies below 7% in Archaic foragers and frequencies over 15% in farmer's phases contemporary to the first contact with Europeans (Larsen, 1997). In prehistoric peoples from Colombia, the prevalence of caries is close to zero in hunter-gatherers that used lithic technology, appears in early farmers and increases in pottery-makers, reaching frequencies of up to 76% (Rodríguez, 2003). These same tendencies have been observed in native modern peoples that had their traditional diets replaced by western ones, during the process of global colonization (Holloway et al., 1963; Mayhall, 1970).

Caselitz (1998) analyzed the historical evolution of caries in 518 human populations of Europe, Asia and America in a wide timeline from the Paleolithic to the present, confirming that during Paleolithic and Mesolithic periods, the hunter-gatherers had less caries and lesions progressed more slowly. Caries indices have increased gradually from Neolithic times, until they reach the high rates observed at the present. Considering only the Holocene (the last 10,000 BC) in the Old World, he observed that the low indices[7] of Mesolithic times remain relatively constant during the Early Neolithic (between the 9th and 5th millennium

---

[6] Agriculture is a set of knowledge and techniques aimed to control the natural environment for production of crops. The transition from the hunting-gathering economy to self-sufficient food production changed radically the human history, promoting a high population growth for food availability, sedentary settlements, new labor division, and changes in the rights of land property that led to a more complex society, with specialists, social classes and centralized government systems.

[7] For his comparisons, Caselitz used a reduced variant of the DMF Index (Decayed Missing Filling Index) applied to archaeological samples, the I-CE (Index of carie-extractio) or DMI (Decay Missing Index – Lukacs, 1996; Pezo & Eggers, 2010; Saunders et al., 1997), calculated as the number of carious teeth added to the number of antemortem toot loss (AMTL) divided by the sum of teeth and sockets observed.

BC), but suffered a dramatic increase of 75% in a short time span of few centuries around 4500 BC. This phenomenon, observed in North Africa, Near East, China and Europe has been attributed to the drastic change in the diet that means the introduction and spread of cereals in the entire antique world (Caselitz, 1998).

In the Mediterranean region, Arabia and India the increase of caries began early between the 7th and 5th millennium BC. In Natufians from the Levant region, the phase of hunter-gatherers (10,500-8300 BC) shows 6.4% of caries frequency whereas Neolithic populations (8300-5500 BC) show 6.7% (Eshed et al., 2006). In the Indo region the caries frequencies range between 1.4-1.8% in the earliest populations, but in the site of Harappa (5000 BP, Pakistan) from the Early Bronze Age[8] the caries frequency is 12% (Lukacs, 1992, 1996) whereas an Iron Age skeletal sample from Oman shows 32.4% (Nelson & Lukacs, 1994) analyzed under the same methods (Fig. 2a). During the Chinese Neolithic, the initial phase Yangshao (7000 – 5000 BP) shows rare evidence of caries (0.04%) and all of them occur in the posterior sector of the mouth. The Longshan period (4500 – 4000 BP) presents caries frequencies of 0.30% and besides, showing caries located in the anterior teeth. The Chinese farming in this epoch was based on domesticated species of millet (*Setaria italica*), broomcorn millet (*Panicum miliaceum*) and rice (*Oryza sativa* – Pechenkina et al., 2002).

The most antique written reference of oral diseases in this region comes from a tablet of clay with cuneiform inscriptions from the lower valley of the Euphrates dated at 5000 BC. The tablet refers to the existence of a "worm" responsible for tooth pain and a recipe for spelling it. More than 3000 years later, in Egypt, the Eber's papyrus, a kind of medical tractate dated around 1550 BC, refers to the existence of gingivitis, pulpitis and dental pain and their treatment using dressings, mouth washers and enchantments (Nikiforouk, 1985). In antique civilizations caries and antemortem teeth loss seemed to be a permanent scourge that obviously must have caused the same physical and psychological suffering it causes nowadays. The first attempts of restorative dentistry have been recorded in Egyptians, Phoenicians, Etruscans and Romans (Asbell, 1948; Harris et al., 1975; Jackson, 1988; Puech, 1995; Teschler-Nichola et al., 1998).

In Europe caries rates are almost stable during the Middle Bronze Age (1600-1200 BC) and increase continuously between 1200 BC and 500 AD. It could mean that the spread of agriculture occurred at least one millennium later than in other Old World regions. A little peak is observed around 750 AD followed by a phase relatively stable during the Middle Age and a second increase, much more dramatic, is observed since the 16th century, and it has reached the highest records in our times (Caselitz, 1998). Examining the proportion of affected individuals per population, Caselitz (1998) observed that during the fifth millennium BC, around one third of individuals were affected with caries. In the Middle and Late Bronze Age (1500-300 BC) the affected proportion of individuals decreases relatively and then rose dramatically to 56% in the 7th century AD. This condition of deterioration remains constant until around 1300 AD when it reaches a new peak. In more

---

[8] In 1820, Christian Thomsen classified the prehistory of Europe in three ages (Cooper Age or Chalcolithic, Bronze Age and Iron Age) based on the analysis of metallic artifacts. Bronze Age was divided into Antique, Middle and Final Bronze Age but dates are different according to the region analyzed. In the Near East bronze appears at the final of the 4th millennium BC, in Greece around 2500 BC, in Persia in 2000 BC, and only about 1800 BC in China (Lull et al., 1991).

recent periods of Modern Age, almost 60% of individuals were affected, and in contemporary times the observations denote global values surpass 95% (Nikiforouk, 1985; Rugg-Gunn & Hackett, 1993; Shafer et al., 1983). These trends have been pointed out in other studies (Moore & Corbet, 1971, 1973, 1975; Roberts & Cox, 2007 – Fig. 2b).

In the American continent caries has been recorded since approximately 7000 BC with relatively high indices that decrease around 5000 BC (Bernal et al., 2007; Caselitz, 1998). A dramatic increase was noticed since 2300 BC. Although we do not have complete dietary inventories for each different period, the high caries rates of the oldest Americans could be related to the consumption of endemic fruits rich in maltodextrines and sugar, such as carob (*Prosopis sp.*) and acacia (*Acacia sp.*). This decrease could be explained by a reorientation in the subsistence activities that turned to marine foraging during the Middle Holocene (around 6000 BP), whereas the highest peak can be clearly related with the summit of agricultural production.

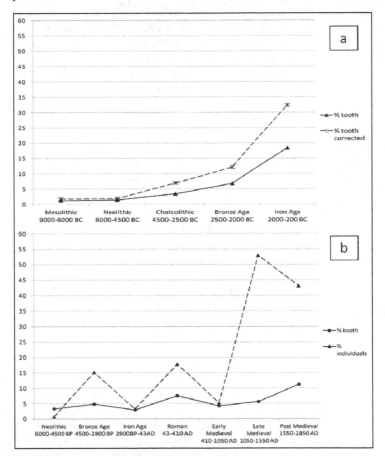

Fig. 2. **Caries trends in the Old World across time.** a) Indus valley civilization sequence, caries frequency versus corrected frequency (Lukacs, 1996). b) Britain sequence, caries frequency versus prevalence (Roberts & Cox, 2007).

In pre-contact America, the consumption of starchy seed-bearing plants like chenopodiaceous, cucurbitaceous, fabaceous, asteraceous (sunflower) has been suggested as the first stage of farming (between 8000-5000 BP) and is related to the first changes in the oral pathological profiles (Bernal et al., 2007; Pezo, 2010; Piperno, 2011). The increase of caries frequency has been attributed mainly (but not exclusively) to maize consumption[9] (*Zea mays* - Larsen et al., 1991; White, 1994) and more specifically to a gradual replacement of popcorn (*indurata* variety), consumed in the earliest periods, for a softer, sweeter and thus more cariogenic, amylaceous maize (*amylacea* or *saccharata* variety) during the second millennium BC (Pezo, 2010; Rodríguez, 2003). However, it is possible that due to the enormous dietary variety derivate from a multiplicity of ecological niches, there are other potentially cariogenic products such as tubercles (wild and cultivated), as well as sweet and sticky fruits (Bernal et al., 2007; Neves & Cornero, 1997; Pezo, 2010).

3.2 Caries: Frequencies and profiles in the last 2000 years

Comparative analyses between Late Antique and Early Medieval populations in Europe show a clear oral health deterioration pattern with high frequencies of caries, abscesses, antemortem tooth loss, alveolar resorption and more severe dental wear in the medieval epochs due to an impoverishment in life conditions after the down of the Western Roman Empire (Belcastro et al., 2007; Manzi et al., 1999; Slaus et al., 2011).

During the Roman Imperial Age (1st-4th centuries AD) caries affects 71.6% of the individuals and 15% of the teeth from Quadrella necropolis (Isernia, Italy). Lesions are more frequent in the posterior teeth and cervical caries are more frequent than occlusal ones. Moreover, occlusal caries decrease with age while cervical ones increase (Bonfiglioli et al., 2003). In general, caries frequencies of Late Antique populations range between 4-15%, whereas in the Early Medieval sites they range between 11.7-17.5% (Slaus et al., 2011). These noticeable differences suggest a drastic change in the dietary habits with a significant increase of carbohydrates in the Early Medieval times.

Historical records state that the typical diet of the middle and low classes in the Western Roman Empire was based on: bread (rich in impurities), porridge of cereals, some pulses, vegetables, olives, some fruits and wine, as well as goats and sheeps. Throughout the Empire diet was quiet homogeneous (Dosi & Schnell., 1990). In the medieval Europe low-class subsistence was based essentially on cereals (the bread represents the 70% of their intake) whereas the protein consumption (meat from hunting or shepherded animals and fresh fish) was low and uncommon (Mazzi, 1981).

The medieval diet of Mediterranean peasants was composed mainly by cereals, specially bread, wheat and barley, pulses (broad beans, peas, lentils, chickpeas), and fruits such as figs, olives, plums, peaches, pine kernels, almonds and grapes (Eclassan et al., 2009). In Britain the most common products were wheat, barley, oats, rye, beans, milk, cheese, eggs, bacon and fowl and the diet of the poor classes was probably restricted to coarse black bread

---

[9] Undoubtedly, corn was one of the most valuable products in the ritual and daily life within Americas. Whereas in Mesoamerica it seems that it has been cultivated almost exclusively (monoculture), in the Andes was only one of the most important crops, consumed in several ways and used to prepare "*chicha*" (maize beer) (Antúnez de Mayolo, 1981; Bonavia, 2008).

(Moore & Corbett, 1973). In Scandinavia, the medieval diet was basically composed of high amounts of salted herring and dried fish, but also barley porridge, turnips, cabbages, dried sour rye bread, sour milk products, some meat, and beer (Varrela, 1991). Only in Spain there was a higher consumption of sugar cane[10] and rice, introduced by the Muslims during almost eight centuries of Iberia occupation (López et al., 2010). In that epoch food was much more abrasive because the flour (milled by millstones) kept some grid that was incorporated to the bread. The cooking or storage techniques using ashes, or consumption of preparations made with unclean flour or non-dehusked grain of hulled cereals such as broomcorn (*Panicum miliaceum*) or barley (*Hordeum vulgare*) were common (Eclassan et al., 2009).

People from medieval French villages of Languedoc from the 13th-14th centuries show caries frequencies of 17.5%, with frequent occlusal and approximal caries (Eclassan et al., 2009). For medieval populations of England and Scotland from the 13th -15th centuries the caries frequency vary between 6.0-7.4% (Kerr et al., 1990; Watt et al., 1997), whereas in medieval sites in Croatia from the 11th-12th centuries the prevalence of caries is 45%, with frequencies or 9.5%, identical to the reported for later sites from the 14th-15th centuries of the same region (Slaus et al., 1997; Vodanovic et al., 2005). In general, Late Medieval populations do not present frequencies significantly higher than Early Medieval populations. It suggests that in a time span of eight centuries, no significant changes in diet occurred (Vodanovic et al., 2005).

Several studies have concluded that the most common locations of caries during the medieval epoch were occlusal and cervical approximal caries, whereas interproximal ones appear rarely (Eclassan et al., 2009; Kerr et al., 1990; Vodanovic et al., 2005; Varrela, 1991; Watt et al., 1997). Meanwhile, around the 10th-11th century, some changes in the location patterns of caries in populations in Continental and Islander Europe are evident. There is a gradual reduction in cervical-approximal caries (CEJ caries[11]) that was more common during the Antique Age, and an increase of occlusal, buccal, and lingual lesions, that have occurred since earlier ages. These data suggest that infantile diet became softer until the final of Middle Age (Lingström & Borrman, 1999; Moore, 1993; Moore & Corbett, 1975; Varrela, 1991; Vodanovic et al., 2005; Watt et al., 1997).

The transition from Middle to Modern Age in Europe was characterized by a remarked increase of flour for bread fabrication and consumption of sugar cane. The possibility of purchasing vegetables and grains in open markets seems to have contributed to the raise of

---

[10] The earliest evidence of domestic sugar cane (8000 BC) comes from New Guinea, Southeast Asia (Sharpe, 1998). After domestication, it spreaded rapidly to southern China, Indochina and India. Sugar cane was taken to Persia during Dario's epoch, where it was discovered by the Macedonian armies in the 4th century BC. Greeks and Romans know it as a "salt from India" and imported it only for medicinal purposes due to its high cost. The crystallized sugar was discovered in India during the Gupta dynasty, around 350 AD. Muslims discovered the sugar when they invaded Persia in 642 AD and spreaded its consumption in Western Europe after they conquered Iberia in the eighth century AD. The first reference about sugar in England, where it was considered a "fine spice", dates from the Crusades epoch in 11th century. In the 12th century, Venice built some colonies near Tyre (modern Lebanon) and began to exports sugar to Europe. Sugar was taken to America in the second trip of Columbus in 1493 (Bernstein, 2009; Parker, 2011).
[11] These lesions have been attributed to physiological compensatory super-eruption of roots subsequent to severe occlusal wear produced by abrasive diets (Eclassan et al., 2009). However, the possible origin related to sweet beverages must be considered (Pezo, 2010; Pezo & Eggers, 2010).

caries and other oral diseases during that time (Bibby, 1990; López et al., 2011). In the first half of the 17th century, Scandinavian populations, with a diet based on marine products show a caries prevalence of about 60% and frequencies of approximately 13% with increases in antemortem tooth loss among the oldest individuals. Carious lesions were most common in the occlusal area, CEJ and interproximal surfaces predominantly in lower molars. In these populations, lesions are uncommon in children but appear earlier in young adults (Lingstrom & Borrman, 1999; Mellquist & Sandberg, 1939; Varrela, 1991).

Since the 17th century, and especially during 18th century, many kinds of foods were brought from America to Europe. Among them are: maize, beans, potatoes, tomatoes, cocoa, coffee and sugar (Prats & Rey, 2003). Although sugar and sugar cane came to the West from India carried by the army of Alexander the Great in 327 BC, the "white sugar" had not became a commercial product until the 7th century. It was largely distributed until the final of 12th century(Bernstein, 2009), but it has only been imported in large scales from America to Europe since 1550 AD when sugar cane plantations increased in Brazil and in the Caribbean islands (Saunders et al., 1997; Parker, 2011). The effect of refined food on caries trends can be observed clearly in Europe during the 18th century and coincides with the increase in the production of refined sugar and the introduction of flour mills.

Populations from the 11th century cemeteries, that were excavated in Britain, Canada and USA show caries frequencies over 35% and a high number of antemortem tooth loss due to caries mostly on inferior molars. For that epoch, changes follow the same trend: cervical lesions (CEJ caries) are less common and more lesions appear in the occlusal surfaces and interproximal contact areas (Moore, 1993; Moore & Corbett, 1975; Saunders et al., 1997).

In the North American colonial diet, meat (pork, beef, and mutton), bread, and vegetables were the staples, and sweet-baked goods were also popular. Maple sugar, maize (used as corn meal flour), pumpkins, and wild fruits were harvested as well. The recipes were all almost the same, and people consumed three meals a day. The use of refined flour for the production of bread and pastries seems to have been very important and bread is still one of the most important items. In addition, the use of corn meal porridge, cooked, sweetened flour mixtures and stewed, sweetened fruits probably contributed to the cariogenicity[12] of the diet (Boyce, 1972; Moore, 1993; Saunders et al., 1997).

However, those remarkable caries increments, occurred during the second half of the 19th century, have been attributed to dramatic increases in the intake of sugar and refined carbohydrates between 1830 and 1880 (Corbett & Moore, 1975; Moore, 1993). Since 1860 the importation of cane caused impressive improvements in per-capita consumption (Saunders et al., 1997). In the 1840 decade England, USA and Canada had an approximate consumption of 30 lb/person. At the end of the century those amounts raised to around 80 lb in England, 60 lb in USA and 50 lbs. in Canada (Boyce, 1972; Saunders et al., 1997). Besides, the introduction of ceramic mills in North America in 1875 (Leung, 1981), produced flours of better quality that favored its industrialization and massive consumption (Boyce, 1972).

---

[12] A cariogenic diet has been defined by the following features: frequent intake of meals with a high content of carbohydrates quickly fermentable (mainly sucrose) with retentive and sticky consistence that produces repetitive lowering of pH values and changes in the ecology of dental plaque. The cariogenic diet produces increase and quicker development of lesions, and location in non-retentive surfaces (Nikiforouk, 1985; Rugg-Gunn & Hackett, 1993).

Caries increase tendency seems to have been constant during the second half of the 19th century and the first half of the 20th century, worldwide. On the other hand, preventive policies against caries did not have considerable effects until the second half of 20th century. France and England were major manufacturers of toothbrushes in 19th century, but they were considered luxury articles and regular tooth brushing was not a widespread practice until after the second half of 19th century (Asbell, 1992).

Since the 1970s a striking decline in caries experiences has been observed throughout industrialized countries (Brunelle & Carlos, 1990; Shafer et al., 1983). This seems to be related to dental treatment and the introduction of fluoride[13] water and toothpaste. Also, the decline in dental caries rates was due to a range of changing social factors that seem to be linked to improvements in general health indicators (**Haugejorden, 1996;** Nikiforouk, 1985; Shaw, 1985). But in emerging countries the situation is the opposite and high caries rates are associated with malnutrition, absence of health services and poor quality of life (Alvarez, 1988; Campodónico et al., 2001; Heredia & Alva, 2005).

3.3 Diet and the "main villain" in the raise of caries throughout human history

The available data indicates that the modern trends on caries increases start simultaneously with permanent growth intake of sucrose during the last two centuries. The hypotheses of an increase in the susceptibility or resistance diminishment by genetic reasons or the installation of a particularly cariogenic flora have not been sufficiently corroborated (De Soet & Laine, 2008; Hassell & Harris, 1995; Shuler, 2001; van Palenstein et al., 1996) while dietary changes seem to be the most reasonable answer. In the modern western world and increasingly in other regions of the globe approximately half of consumed calories comes from carbohydrates and almost half of it is sucrose.

Until recently, several populations living in isolated areas of the world kept their ancestral ways of life (for instance, many African tribes, Inuits, South American Indians, Melanesian, Polynesian) under conditions of perfect adaptation to their environments and diets (Donnelly et al., 1977; Mayhall, 1977; Pedersen, 1971; Schamschula et al., 1980; Walker & Hewlett, 1990). Bacteriologic analyses of their dental plaques, although not extensive, show cariogenic species, but those individuals are still developing few or no caries. Otherwise, when those populations were acculturated or simply replaced their traditional diet for an "occidental refined diet", they started to develop progressively destructive caries patterns.

The case of the British colony of Tristan da Cunha, a volcanic island in the South Atlantic, described several times since 1817, is famous. Until the Second World War their diet was based on fish and potatoes (from their own production) and they were visited by a ship once or twice a year. Despite their poor hygiene, the majority of them were free of caries. When the war started many factories and military stations were built on the island deeply changing the lifestyle of the population and facilitating the importation of other foodstuff.

---

[13] The fluoride contained in water has been recognized as a control factor of caries but high amounts of fluoride can produce recognizable enamel defects that usually involve a pattern of opacity named fluorosis (Fejerskov et al., 1994). Fluorosis has been reported in archaeological series related to consumption of phreatic waters from wells (Pezo, 2010; Valdivia, 1980).

The deterioration of their oral conditions was evident in the beginning of the 1950's. In 1962, when the volcanic activity obliged inhabitants to evacuate towards England, more than 40 % of their teeth were affected by caries or had been destroyed. The most notable change in life conditions of those individuals was diet, with a decrease in the consumption of potatoes and a compensatory consumption of sugar. It is estimated that the daily consumption of sugar rose from 1.8 g. in 1938 to 150 g. in 1966, three years after their return from England. On the other hand, under equivalent conditions, older people did not seem to be as resistant as their descendents (Holloway et al., 1963). Data that confirms this tendency have also been reported for populations from developing countries (Corraini et al., 2009; Ismail et al., 1997; Petersen & Kaka, 1999; Petersen & Razanamihaja, 1996).

Whereas the role of sugar as the main "villain" in the caries etiology seems to be evident, it is disputable if starches play a similar role (Tayles et al., 2000, 2009). By their slow accumulation in dental plaque and slower oral digestion, starch could have a relative low cariogenicity and its importance as a factor of caries depends on the simultaneous intake with sucrose as well as the frequency of its consumption (Frostell et al., 1967). Thus, starch has been defined as "co-cariogenic", especially when it is gelatinized by thermal effect (Grenby, 1997). The gelatinization of starch[14] seems to be the determining factor of its cariogenicity, because in general, only gelatinized starches are susceptible to enzymatic breakage (through salivary or bacterial pocesses) to produce highly cariogenic molecules (Grenby, 1997; Lingström et al., 2000). Nevertheless, the necessary temperature for starch gelatinization surpasses 80°C in most of the cases.

In this sense, the invention of pottery (the earliest pottery appeared in the Samara region of South-Eastern Russia about 7000 BC – Anthony, 2007), its spread and common use for storage and cooking could have been a significant trigger for the raise of caries markers before the popularization of refined sucrose consumption. Until the introduction of pottery, other cooking methods were employed around the world, but those methods would hardly result in gelatinization of starche[15] (Antúnez de Mayolo, 1981; Pezo, 2010; Wrangham, 2009). The refinement and cooking of carbohydrates produce an increase in their retentive and sticky capacity the tooth surface leading to slower clearance times. For instance, bread starch shows higher clearance times than starches from potatoes or rice (Grenby, 1997; Lingström et al., 2000).

According to some authors, cooking can eliminate some protective agents (against the caries) of certain foodstuff. The Bantu of Africa show an increase in caries frequency after the adoption of a colonial diet. The amount of cereals and sugar were the same, but they

---

[14] During the process of cooking food, the starch granules are disintegrated by heat and mechanical forces. Eventually the liberation of the molecules in a process named gelatinization occurs. The temperature and water-starch proportion necessary to gelatinization are very variable in accordance to each distinct starches. For instance, the temperature for rice gelatinization ranges between 85-111°C with a proportion water-starch of 2.0-0.75 and ranges between 65-90°C for maize starch (Lingström et al., 2000; Donald, 2004).

[15] These traditional methods include: a) the use of heated stones for boiling liquids within pumpkins and squashes; they were also used to roast meat and vegetables by direct contact or placed along with the food into the underground ovens covered with earth; b) roasting by direct contact with fire (as for mollusks or turtles); c) roasting of meat and vegetables wrapped in leaves or packed in bamboo canes over wood grills, among others.

were refined for cooking. In this case, by *in vitro* studies, caries increase was attributed to the absence of phytate, an organic phosphate contained in cereals that can be extracted easily by boyling (Bowen, 1994; Osborn & Noriskin, 1937). Thus, the softer texture and the elimination of "protective factors" through cooking increase cariogenicity.

On the other hand, there are some foods that inhibit the formation of caries. Diets rich in meat lead to low caries frequencies due to the fatty acids' antibacterial power and their capacity to reduce the adherence of plaque on dental surfaces. The intake of dairy products and fish (foods rich in calcium and casein that can increase urea concentration) modifies pH values and the quantity of salivary production, inhibiting the formation of dental plaque. Finally, a food rich in polyphenols (such as cacao, coffee and tea) inhibits the bacterial metabolism and stimulates the salivary secretion representing, thus, another mechanism of caries prevention (Bowen, 1994; Touger-Decker & Loveren, 2003).

Caries frequencies of only 0.3% - 0.6%, with prevalence of around 4% have been reported for the Inuit from Angmagssalik (East Greenland), isolated until 1884 and with a diet based on meat and fish, almost without carbohydrates. These observations are in accordance with prevalences of 0.4% - 2.5% and frequencies of 0.08% - 0.35% (mainly little carious lesions in molar fissures) in craniums of ancient Inuits and are strikingly different from that observed in neighboring populations with access to sugar and cereals (Mayhall, 1977; Pedersen 1947, 1952).

Little changes in the type of carbohydrate, texture, mode of conservation and preparing of meals can produce utterly different caries experiences (Molnar, 1972; Rodríguez, 2003; Turner, 1979). In Paleolithic and Mesolithic populations it is common to observe the effects of an abrasive and non-refined diet. The ancient people show an aggressive dental wear that frequently surpasses the speed of development of little aggressive carious lesion, producing an exposure of the pulp chamber with abscesses formation and consequent tooth loss (Fig. 3). In Neolithic populations the change to better processed diets gradually leads to a low wear of masticatory surfaces that is another factor why the occlusal caries could have developed earlier. This competitive relation between dental wear[16] and caries has been also observed in fishermen from the South American Pacific coast, Dutch sailors from 18th -19th centuries and in other populations with marine subsistence (Milner, 1984; Maat & Van der Velde, 1987; Pezo & Eggers, 2010). Finally, dental wear is a factor that can distort the real perception of caries experience in several populations with abrasive diet.

However, there are also some cases that have reported a positive correlation between caries and dental wear, as observed in Mesolithic populations from Portugal and Sicily (Meiklejhon et al., 1988; Lubell et al., 1994) where the consumption of honey, figs and sweet fruits accelerates the installation of caries in attrition surfaces. This phenomenon has also been noticed for the Pecos from South West -USA during the Archaic Period (4000-1000 BC) with caries prevalence of 14% and pulp chamber exposure as the main cause of tooth loss (Larsen, 1997). Thus, the cariogenic capacity of natural sugars contained in honey and sweet

---

[16] Dental wear is related to the physical consistence of food, the storage ways and the technology used in their processing. Analyses of coprolites (fossilized faeces) have shown some abrasive material such as phytolithes (microscopic silica structures contained in certain plant organs), seeds, little bone fragments and oxalate calcium crystals from some species (Larsen, 1997; Pearsall, 2000). Besides, historical and ethnographical data from several regions of the world describe the ingestion of abrasives such as ashes and clays as part of the meals (Antúnez de Mayolo, 1981; Indriati & Buikstra, 2001; Rodríguez, 2003).

fruits such as carob, figs, and prickly pear might not be understated because they have been noticed as responsible for the high caries prevalence in some populations (Bernal et al., 2007; Nelson et al., 1999; Neves & Cornero, 1997; Pezo, 2010).

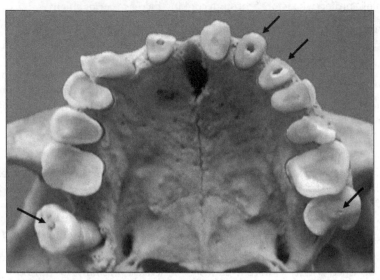

Fig. 3. **Competitive relation between caries and dental wear in an individual with abrasive diet.** Carious lesions almost eliminated through dental wear in molars, and pulp chamber exposure due to severe wear in anterior teeth.

Finally, drastic climatic changes, complex social processes, and wars can lead to resource searching by strategies considered "regressive", as well as technological innovations (Hillson, 2001; Molnar, 1972). Walker & Erlandson (1986) studied caries and dietary changes in Santa Rosa Island (Santa Barbara Channel, South California), during a time span from 4000 to 400 BP, observing that in the first 1500 years predominantly terrestrial products such as starchy roots and tubers were exploited, and later they readapted their subsistence strategies to marine sources dropped from 13.3 to 6.3% in the caries frequencies, following the reduction in carbohydrates intake.

On the other hand, there are some exceptions about the correspondence between agriculture and caries. Several groups of modern farmers with a diet based almost exclusively on starch rich foods such as taro, sweet potato, and manioc, show low caries frequencies (Barmes et al., 1970; Baume 1969). In populations from Eastern Asia, the consumption of rice, despite their frequency, has produced low caries experiences (Tayles et al., 2000). Other especially high values of caries in populations with hunter-gatherers technology have been attributed to the consumption of cariogenic species traded with neighbor farmers[17] (Lukacs, 1990; Walker & Hewlett, 1990).

---

[17] African pigmies (Aka, Mbuti, Efe) traded meat and honey with the Bantu, who provided back manioc, maize, nuts, rice and plantains. In these hunter-gatherers honey is an important dietary source during great part of the year (Walker & Hewlett, 1990).

As we can see, the historical evaluation of caries allows us to recognize some trends and recurrences in prevalences, frequencies and patterns. Although in general it is possible to identify some critical variables such as the excessive consumption of refined sucrose or gelatinized starches as etiological agents, there are many other socio-historical factors, specific for each population, that must be considered before generalizing about the complex relationship between caries and subsistence pattern.

4. Key factors related to caries prevalence in human populations: Physiological or cultural factors?

Much of the studies carried out in hunter-gatherers and farmers from different latitudes and temporal periods have stated a particular trend: women show higher caries prevalences than men (Larsen et al., 1991; Lukacs, 1992, 1996, 2008, 2011; Luckacs & Largaespada, 2006; Milner, 1984; Rodríguez, 2003; Walker & Hewlett, 1990). This phenomenon suggests two possible, not necessarily excluding, explanations: a) there is a major constitutional predisposition in females to caries; b) the differences are culturally regulated.

Clinical researches of the last decades have revealed that physiological differences between sexes have an important indirect impact on oral ecology. The saliva's chemical composition and flow are modified in various manners according to hormonal fluctuations associated with puberty, menstruation, and pregnancy. These processes lead to a much more cariogenic oral environment in females than in males. Estrogen levels are positively correlated with caries rates whereas androgens do not affect them (Lukacs & Largaespada, 2006). Experimental and clinical studies show that pregnancy reduces the buffer capacity of saliva and produces xerostomy that promotes bacterial growth, increasing the susceptibility to caries (Bergdahl, 2000; Dowd, 1999; Lukacs & Largaespada, 2006; Salvolini et al., 1998; Valdéz et al., 1993).

From an evolutionary perspective, it has been suggested that the increase of fertility that accompanied the sedentary lifestyle and the adoption of agriculture had a significant effect on the increase in caries rates worldwide (Lukacs, 2008). The classic proverb "a tooth per child" expresses the traditional idea that pregnancy results in a deterioration of oral health along with a weakening in the tooth structure and subsequent caries development and tooth loss (Lukacs, 2011; Lukacs & Largaespada, 2006). However, although there is evidence of increased periodontal inflammation in women during pregnancy, tooth loss due to pregnancy is more controversial (Larsen et al., 1991; Lukacs, 2011).

From the same point of view, the fact that much more males than females show high caries frequencies have been interpreted as a cultural mechanism of adaptation, in which young men are selectively buffered from malnutrition, through the exposition to higher amounts of cariogenic foods (Slaus et al. 1997). However, women usually show more severe nutritional stress markers, such as frequent enamel hypoplasias, less intervals between defects and more frequent tooth growth disruptions (King et al., 2005).

Among other "constitutional" reasons argued for this repetitive higher prevalence of caries in women, the earlier eruption of the female dentition (that exposes the teeth for longer time), has been also mentioned. This assertion, however, has not demonstrated strong correlation with caries prevalence (Larsen, 1997). On the other hand, if the reasons were strictly physiological, then differences between men and women should be universal, but in general there are many clinical and archaeological examples that suggest the existence of other factors involved (Powell, 1988; White, 1994). So, despite the plausible possibility that women show a higher intrinsic physiologic susceptibility towards caries than man, the caries experience is behaviorally mediated.

It has been observed that in populations where caries are higher in women, there is usually a differentiated consumption of foods: men consuming more meat and women consuming more carbohydrates. Contemporary foragers populations show that men, responsible for getting the protein, consumes more amounts from the meat that they hunted, whereas women, responsible for vegetables gathering, and food preparation, consume more carbohydrates during their activities (Walker & Erlandson, 1986; Walker & Hewlett, 1990). Furthermore, men eat some few "big" meals along the journey, whereas women eat several "little" ones, causing more exposition to caries (Gustafsson et al., 1953; Rugg-Gunn & Edgar, 1984; Wrangham, 2009).

Interestingly, the differences between men and women are much more subtle among farmers. However, these slight differences also seem to be related more to cultural than constitutional factors. The Bantu show high caries prevalence in accordance to their considerable intake of carbohydrates and men have higher frequencies than women (9.1% versus 7.1% - Walker & Hewlett, 1990). The same happens in some populations from South American Andes where the carious lesions (mainly cervical ones) are much more frequent in males that preserve the ancestral habit of coca leaf chewing (Pando, 1988). This pattern has also been observed in archaeological samples (Indriati & Buikstra, 2001; Langsjöen, 1996; Pezo & Eggers, 2010; Valdivia, 1980). In Andean and Amazonian populations, it was observed higher prevalence in women who are responsible for chewing maize and manioc as a part of preparing fermentable beverages (*chicha, masato, kiki* - Larsen, 1997; Pezo & Eggers, 2010).

On the other hand, we must consider the effect of social differences in the patterns of food consumption in stratified societies (Cucina & Tiesler, 2003; Gagnon, 2004; Sakashita et al., 1997). There is growing evidence suggesting that members from different social classes, consuming different foods, tend to have different patterns of dental disease. In Copán (Honduras) and Lamanai (Belize), during the Classic Maya Period, elites show lower prevalence of caries than ordinary people. Among low-status burials, there are significantly more caries than in high-status individuals. It was also observed, through an isotopic study, that low-status individuals eat mainly carbohydrates (maize). Stable isotopes studies confirmed that low-status individuals eat mainly carbohydrates (maize), whereas elite individuals consumed much less maize and had easy access to animal protein, and in general, a much varied and cariostatic diet (Reed, 1994). Contrarily, among citizens and slaves from Yin-Shang period (Anyang, China) oral diseases were significantly higher in citizens' samples (Sakashita et al., 1997). High-status individuals from the Peruvian North Coast (Late Formative, 400-1 BC) do not show more caries than their low-status contemporary ones (Gagnon, 2004).

Comparisons between social classes show contradictory results in medieval Europe. Individuals from all social classes, buried around the Westerhuss church (Sweden), do not show differences in caries prevalence that suggest similar diets independently of social status (Swardstedt, 1966). In Zalavár (Hungary), however, high class individuals linked to the castle show significantly lower caries frequencies (6.4%) than ordinary village people (12.1% - Fryer, 1984). In post-medieval Europe caries tends to affect more the opulent class than the poor class due to the regular consumption of sweet foods. Since that epoch caries has been perceived as an occupational disease among bakers and confectioners (Götze et al., 1986; Kainz & Sonnabend, 1983). Historical records of the meals served for the Spanish royalty of the 18th century included meat broths and stews from hunted and breeding animals that contained wine, sugar and cinnamon, while bread was the usual side order. The last part of each main meal was the sweet dessert that included cakes, creams, sugar coated donuts, fruit tartlets, cookies, jelly, fruits with syrup, dates, pomegranates, nuts, hazelnuts, and figs. The Spanish royalty usually consumed chocolate that was the unique food permitted during the penitence days (Pérez Samper, 2003).

From these information we can infer that, although it is true that high caries frequencies are associated to poverty and a restrict diet (rich in carbohydrates and poor in animal protein), it is also true that in some periods better economic conditions facilitated a more frequent intake of food, increasing also the amount of cariogenic substratum for certain sub-groups of the population. Other socio-economical factors must be carefully considered; among them, the unfavorable conditions of dental structure development due to malnutrition and hypocalcification that turns tooth much more vulnerable to caries attack (Alvarez, 1988; Campodónico et al., 2001; Heredia & Alva, 2005; Hollister & Weintraub, 1993). Finally, enamel defects, more common in emerging countries due to nutritional stress, can facilitate the development of carious lesions under the presence of cariogenic diets (Nikiforou & Fraser, 1981).

5. The new research agenda on the historical relation between caries and food

The main objective of the study of caries and other dental diseases from the anthropological point of view is to recognize long term dietary changes related to historical events, with the purpose of understanding the rise of civilization as an integrated process that articulates not only new subsistence patterns and technologies but also new forms of relationship among human beings.

Bioanthropological literature offers several comparative studies of caries among groups with known subsistence patterns and social organization that indicates that dental diseases are less frequent or do not appear in hunter-gatherers, whereas they are more frequent and variable in farmers (Table 2). However, there is not simple or universal explanation for patterns of changes in caries frequencies during human history (Tayles et al., 2000, 2009).

The relationship between caries and agriculture is based on the assumption of an increase of carbohydrate in the diet and the supposition that all these carbohydrates are cariogenic. This assumption has led many scholars to infer, solely based on the increase of caries rates, the adoption of agriculture. However, the lower caries rates observed in Asiatic rice-eating farmers contradicts this assertion (Tayles et al., 2009). On the other hand, there are ethnographic records of a great variety of groups that took advantage of diverse subsistence strategies combining foods from hunting and gathering (terrestrial and/or marine), with vegetables from gathering and farming in different proportions (Hillson, 2001). These groups can not be classified into those two "hermetic" categories (hunter-gatherers and farmers). During the human history many societies show different civilizatory trajectories and "wide spectrum" diets.

Despite, the "typical" frequencies for each type of diet have been used in bioanthropology to infer subsistence and social organization in groups with unknown dietary record[18] (Lukacs, 1992, 1996; Turner, 1978, 1979; Ubelaker, 2000), the use of "simple" caries indices and frequencies have showed limitations. These difficulties arise because of the superposition and non-specificity of the "typical" ranges and the consequent problem of classifying populations with mixed subsistence strategies or developing stages of agricultural subsistence (Godoy,2005; Hillson, 2001; Lukacs, 1992, 1996). In addition, there is a clear association between age and caries experience that is difficult to evaluate in archaeological populations. In living peoples caries progress with the age, and the proportion of teeth affected by coronal or root caries increase with age (Luan et al., 1989; Matthesen et al., 1990). In general, caries experience can be very variable among individuals, with many or few caries per individual, a situation that can obscure the perception of caries frequencies in whole populations.

Because of the fragmentary nature of the archaeological material the loss of information regarding the number of individuals affected in the population and the number of lesions in lost teeth (*antemortem* and *postmortem*[19]) is inevitable. Thus, since it is likely that some teeth lost antemortem should have been lost due to carious lesions, the resultant rate can be produce an under-estimative of the real caries experience of an individual or group. On the other hand, we do not know how many teeth were lost due to caries or other conditions such as trauma and periodontal disease (Carranza, 1986; Lukacs, 2007). Besides that, it is difficult to know how many teeth were present in the lost maxillary segments. For those reasons, modern caries indices such as DMFT or DMFS are unsuitable for bioarchaeological research. Also, diagenetic changes and variable preservation of skeletal series can obscure genuine differences or similarities between sites, making problematic any inter-observer comparisons (Hillson, 2001; Wesolowski, 2006).

The caries rates regularly used in bioanthropology (Duyar & Erdal, 2003; Hillson, 2001; Moore y Corbett, 1971; Lukacs, 1992, 2007; Powell, 1985; Saunders et al., 1997; Watt et al., 1997;) for being numeric, basically count the number of lesions creating a false perception that high frequencies, prevalences or caries indices, correspond to an increase of agricultural development. Furthermore, these rates do not discriminate between the type, severity or exact location of the lesions, which can be much more informative about a diet's cariogenicity. Individuals with carious lesions of different depth and location can have similar caries rates. This fact can obscure the interpretation of caries experience among populations. For instance, a young adult from a group A with two occlusal lesions that affects only enamel has the same numeric index as another young adult from a group B that

---

[18] Evaluating populations with known diets, Turner (1979) defined ranges of characteristics frequencies for each type of subsistence: 0%-5.3% for hunter-gatherers, 0.44% - 10.3% for mixed economies, and 2.2% - 26.9% for farmers.

[19] Approximately 15% of teeth are lost during the process of human remains recovery. These sockets are difficult to be considered for caries indexes because lost teeth could, or could not, have been affected by caries (Larsen, 1997; Pezo, 2010; Saunders et al., 1997).

suffers from two interproximal lesions that affect dentin and pulp. Although they have the same caries frequency and/or index it is possible that their diets are quite different (Fig. 4).

 Pezo & Eggers (2010) employed several dental paleopathology markers to infer past diets in four groups with different stages of agricultural development inhabiting the Peruvian North Coast and observed a paradox overlap of the simple caries frequencies and DMI that did not correspond to technological and social changes of the different epochs. In a more detailed analysis it was observed an increase in the "speed of development" of caries and a gradual change in the caries location from occlusal to extra-occlusal caries, in accordance to the expected for more cariogenic diets associated with the adoption of new vegetal products and new processing technologies that accompanied the agricultural intensification. Sweet fruits and two maize types introduced in different epochs produced totally different caries patterns. In the later period, near to the European contact, when farming technologies reached their maximum apogee, besides carious lesions and other conditions inherent of an agricultural diet, typical culturally inflicted lesions appear: those produced by coca leaf chewing and maize beer or "*chicha*" beverage.

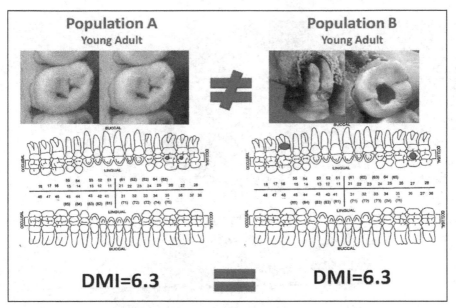

Fig. 4. **The problem of "simple" caries frequencies and indices in Bioanthropology.** In archaeological samples similar indices do not necessarily correspond to similar dietary conditions and comparable caries patterns.

These results, lead us to conclude that the use of caries indices like DMI or the record of simple caries frequencies are insufficient in reflecting known differences in agricultural development because they do not allow one to discriminate between different degrees of cariogenicity of a diet (Fig. 5). Caries depth and location are better markers to evaluate cariogenicity in past populations. The most accurate indicators are dentine caries and extra-occlusal lesions. Occlusal caries are informative, but can be eliminated by intense dental wear (pulp exposures due to dental wear must then be subtracted from the total number of carious lesions). Other comparisons along the time have confirmed an increase of the depth of lesions and more affected dental surfaces, related to the introduction of more cariogenic foods (Bonfiglioli et al., 2003; Hillson, 2001, Godoy, 2005; Pechenkina et al., 2002; Sakashita et al., 1997).

Then, the new challenge of oral paleopathology is to determine the impact of farming of different kinds of crops in different parts of the world by the observation of caries depth and location patterns associated with different diets. Rather than a particular indicator, the "ideal method" for paleodietary reconstruction with oral pathology is the characterization of specific "paleopathological models" produced by the integration of caries, periodontal disease and dental wear patterns obtained through the maximum possible number of markers. Caries depth and location as well as other oral conditions need to be considered in the context of oral ecology. Only an integrative analysis, relying also on as much archaeological data[20] (concerning the contextual social conditions) and bioanthropological evidence as possible can result in more reliable reconstructions of ancient diet.

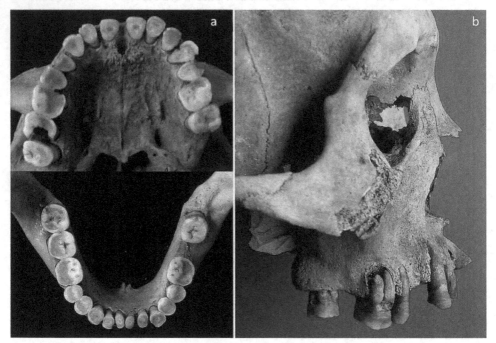

Fig. 5. **Pathological profiles in archaeological samples from the Central Andean Coast.** a) Fisherman with incipient agriculture (around 2400 BC). b) Fully developed farmer with coca leaf chewing habit (around 1300 AD).

---

[20] The methods commonly used for paleodietary reconstruction are: a) the identification of botanical and zoological macro-remains from excavations; b) the physico-chemical analyses (stable isotopes and traces) in bones; c) the identification of botanical micro-remains (phytoliths and starch granules) from dental calculus, coprolites and artifacts (Fry, 2006; Pearsall, 2000).

Population	Frequency (%)	Subsistence pattern
Hunter-gatherers (Turner, 1979)	**0 – 5.3**	
Oklahoma-USA, Fourche Maline, Archaic (Powell, 1985)	0.07	
Cis-Baikal-Siberia, Neolithic Kitoy (Lieverse et al., 2007)	0.23	
Patagonia, NW-MZ Final Late Holocene (Bernal et al., 2007)	3.30	Hunter-gatherers
Patagonia, NW-MZ Early Late Holocene (Bernal et al., 2007)	5.19	
Central Brazil, Paleoindian (Neves & Cornero, 1997)	9.00	
Portugal, Mesolithic (Lubell et al., 1994)	14.30	
Mixed diet (Turner, 1979)	**0.4 – 10.3**	
Alaska, Esquimos pre-contact (Keenleyside, 1998)	<0.05	
Brazilian Shellmound, Middle Holocene (Okumura & Eggers, 2005)	0.40	
Northern Chile (3500–2000 BC) (Kelley et al., 1991)	0.60	Fishermen
Patagonia, NE-RN Middle Late Holocene (Bernal et al., 2007)	0.95	
Alaska, Ipiutak pre-contact (Costa, 1980)	14.40	
Gran Canaria, coastal mounds (Delgado et al., 2006)	6.20	
Early Hawaians (Keene, 1986)	9.80	Fisher-gardeners
Peruvian Coast, Early Formative (Pezo & Eggers, 2010)	21.60	
Farmers (Turner, 1979)	**2.2 – 26.9**	
Portugal, Neolithic (Lubell et al., 1994)	3.10	
China, Ying Shang period (Sakashita et al., 1997)	3.45	
Pakistan, Harappa-Bronze Age (Lukacs, 1992)	6.80	
Turkey, Bizantines 13 th century (Caglar et al., 2007)	6.80	
Florida-USA, Early Mission 1600-1680 (Larsen et al., 2007)	7.40	
Georgia-USA, Early Mission 1600-1680 (Larsen et al., 2007)	7.60	
England, Roman 43-410 AD (Roberts & Cox, 2007)	7.50	
Patagonia, CW-SJFLH Late Holocene (Bernal et al., 2007)	10.17	
Sweden, 17 th century (Lingström & Borrman, 1999)	12.00	
Northern Chile, Maitas (Kelley et al., 1991)	14.40	Farmers
Gran Canaria-inland caves (Delgado et al., 2006)	15.70	
Oman, Iron Age (Nelson & Lukacs, 1994)	18.00	
Peruvian Coast, Middle Formative (Pezo & Eggers, 2010)	21.73	
Peruvian Coast, Epiformative (Pezo & Eggers, 2010)	20.67	
Peruvian Coast, Late Intermediate Period (Pezo & Eggers, 2010)	22.07	
Florida-USA, Late Mission 1680-1700 (Larsen et al., 2007)	24.40	
Texas-USA, Confederate Veterans (Denseizer & Baker, 2004)	24.40	
High Canada, 19th century (Saunders et al., 1997)	35.95	
Northern Chile, Quitor-5 (Kelley et al., 1991)	48.10	

Table 2. Caries frequencies and subsistence patterns among past populations

Comparing peoples living in the same place at different times or groups living in different sites at the same time is more useful and informative than studying an isolated site or population. Statistical analyses, although necessary for the depuration of more important information, must not disregard qualitative analyses. A permanently pending agenda is the refinement of methods and the increase of epidemiological studies in traditional non-Occidentalized groups that can be useful for a better contextualization of future bioarchaeological studies. These research avenues would allow a much better contextualization of future bioarchaeological work. Last but not least, the better knowledge of our past diets will certainly make us better cope with the future of food production and its ecological and health consequences.

6. Acknowledgments

The authors wish to thank Adriana Andrade for the text revision, Maria Mestriner and Suely Praty from the *Biblioteca da Faculdade de Odontologia da Universidade de São Paulo (USP)*, Walter Neves from Laboratório de Estudos Evolutivos Humanos IBUSP, and the support of FAPESP: 2011/503399 and CNPq-bolsa de produtividade.

7. References

Aiello, L.C. & Wheeler, P. (1995). The expensive-tissue hypothesis: The brain and the digestive system in human and primate evolution. *Current Anthropology* 36: 199-221.

Alvarez, J.O. (1988). Chronic malnutrition, dental caries, and tooth exfoliation in Peruvian children aged 3-9 years. *American Journal of Clinic Nutrition* 48:368-72.

Antúnez de Mayolo, S. (1981). *La nutrición en el antiguo Perú*. Ed. Banco Central de Reserva del Perú. Lima.

Anthony, D.W. (2007). *The Horse, the Wheel, and Language*. Princeton University Press, New Jersey.

Asbell, M.B. (1948). Specimens of the dental art in ancient Phoenicia (5th-4th century B.C). *Bulletin of the History of Medicine* 22 (6): 812-821.

Asbell, M.B. (1992) Research in dental caries in the United States: 1820–1920. *Compendium of Continuing Education in Dentistry* 14:792–798.

Baume, L.J. (1969). Caries prevalence and caries intensity among 12,344 school children of French Polynesia. *Archives of Oral Biology* 14 (2): 181-205.

Barmes, D.E., Adkins B.L. & Schamschula, R.G. (1970). Etiology of caries in Papúa-New Guinea: Associations in soil, food and water. *Bulletin World Health Organization* 43: 769-784.

Belcastro, G., Rastelli, E., Mariotti, V., Consiglio. C., Facchini, F. & Bonfiglioli, B. (2007). Continuity or discontinuity of the life-style in central Italy during the Roman Imperial Age-Early Middle Ages transition: Diet, health, and behavior. *American Journal of Physical Anthropology* 132:381–394.

Bermúdez de Castro, J.M., Arsuaga, J.L. & Pérez, P.J. (1997). Interproximal grooving in the Atapuerca SH hominid dentitions. *American Journal of Physical Anthropology* 102, 369e376.

Bernal, V., Novellino, P., Gonzalez, P. & Pérez, I. (2007). Role of wild plant foods among Late Holocene hunter-gatherers from central and north Patagonia (South America):

An approach from dental evidence. *American Journal of Physical Anthropology* 133:1047–1059.

Bartsiokas, A. & Day, M.H. (1993). Lead poisoning and dental caries in the Broken Hill hominid. *Journal of Human Evolution* 24 (3), 243-249.

Bergdahl, M. (2000). Salivary flow and oral complaints in adult dental patients. *Community Dentistry and Oral Epidemiology* 28:59–66.

Bernstein, W. (2009). *A Splendid Exchange: How Trade Shaped the World*. Atlantic Books, London.

Bibby, B.G. (1990). *Food and the Teeth*. Vantage Press, New York.

Bonavia, D. (2008). *El maíz, su origen, su domesticación y el rol que ha cumplido en el desarrollo de la cultura*. Fondo Editorial de la Universidad San Martín de Porras. Lima.

Bonfiglioli, B., Brasili, P. & Belcastro, M.G. (2003). Dento–alveolar lesions and nutritional habits of a Roman Imperial age population (1st–4th c. AD): Quadrella (Molise, Italy). *Homo, Journal of Comparative Human Biology* 54: 36–56.

Bowen, W.H. (1994). Food components and caries. *Advances in Dental Research* 8(2): 215-220.

Boyce, G. (1972). *Hutton of Hastings*. Mika and Mika, Belleville, Ontario.

Boydstun, S., B., Trinkaus, E. & Vandermeersch, B. (1988). Dental caries in the Qafzeh 3 early modern human (abstract). *American Journal of Physical Anthropology* 75, 188–189.

Brennan, M.U. (1991). Health and disease in the Middle and Upper Paleolithic of southwestern France: a bioarcheological study. Ph.D. Thesis. New York University

Brothwell, D.R. (1963). The macroscopic dental pathology of some earlier human populations. In: Brothwell, D.R. (Ed.), *Dental Anthropology*. pp. 271-288. Pergamon Press, Oxford.

Brunelle, J.A. & Carlos, J.P. (1990) Recent Trends in Dental Caries in U.S. Children and the Effect of Water Fluoridation. Journal of Dental Research 69, Special Issue: 723-727.

Buikstra, J. & Beck, L. (Eds.). (2006). *Bioarchaeology. The contextual analysis of human remains*. Academic Press. Elsevier, London.

Caglar, E., Kuscu, O., Sandalli, N. & Ari, I. (2007). Prevalence of dental cáries and tooth wear in a Byzantine population (13th c. A.D.) from northwest Turkey. *Archives of Oral biology* 52: 1136-1145.

Campillo, D. (2001). *Introducción a la Paleopatología*. Bellaterra Arqueología, Barcelona.

Campodónico, C., Pineda, M., Chein, S., Benavente, L. & Ventocilla, M. (2001). El estado nutricional como riesgo para desarrollar caries en niños menores de cinco años de edad. *Odontología Sanmarquina* Vol.1 (7). Date of Access: 15 set 2011, Available from: http://sisbib.unmsm.edu.pe/bvrevistas/odontologia/2001_n7/estado_nutri.htm

Carbonell, E. (Ed.) (2005) *Homínidos: las primeras ocupaciones de los continentes*. Editorial Ariel, Barcelona.

Carranza, F. (1986). *Periodontología clínica de Glickman*. Editoral Interamericana, México DF.

Cartmill, M. (1993) *A View to a Death in the Morning: Hunting and Nature through History*. Harvard University Press, Cambridge.

Caselitz, P. (1998). Caries ancient plague of humankind. In: *Dental Anthropology. Fundamentals, Limits, and Prospects*. Alt, K.W.; Rösing, F.W. & Teschler-Nicola M. (Eds.). pp. 203-226. Springer, Wien, New York.

Clement, A.J. (1956). Caries in the South African ape-man: some examples of undoubted pathological authenticity believed to be 800000 years old. *British Dental Journal* 101: 4-7.

Clement, A.J. (1958). The antiquity of caries. *British Dental Journal* 104(4):115-122.

Cohen, M. & Armelagos, G. (1984). Paleopathology at the origins of agriculture: editor's summation. In: Cohen, M. & Armelagos, G. (Eds). *Paleopathology at the origins of agriculture*. pp. 581–601. Academic Press, Orlando.

Roberts, C. & Cox, M. (2007). The impact of economic intensification and social complexity on human health in Britain from 6000 BP (Neolithic) and the introduction of farming to the Mid-nineteenth century AD. In: Cohen, M. & Crane-Kramer, M.M. (Eds). *Ancient Health: Skeletal Indicators of Agricultural and Economic Intensification*. pp.149-163. University Press of Florida, Gainesville.

Corraini, P., Baelum, V., Pannuti, C.M., Pustiglioni, A.N., Romito, G.A. & Pustiglioni, F.E. (2009). Tooth loss prevalence and risk indicators in an isolated population of Brazil. *Acta Odontologica Scandinavica* 67: 297–303.

Costa, R.L. (1980). Age, sex, and ante-mortem loss of teeth in prehistoric Eskimo skeletal samples from Point Hope and Kodiak Island, Alaska. *American Journal of Physical Anthropology* 53: 579-587.

Crovella, S. & Ardito, G. (1994). Frequencies of oral pathologies in a sample of 767 non-human primates. *Primates* 35, 2: 225-230.

Cucina, A.; Tiesler, V. & Sierra, T. (2003). Sex Differences in oral pathologies at the Late Classic Maya Site of Xcambó, Yucatán1. *Dental Anthropology* 16 (2): 45-51.

Danzeiser, H. & Baker, J.E. (2004). Dental health of elderly Confederate Veterans: Evidence from the Texas State Cemetery. *American Journal of Physical Anthropology* 124:59–72.

Delgado-Darias, T., Velasco-Vázquez, J., Arnay-De La Rosa, M. & González-Reimers E. (2005). Dental caries among the pre-Hispanic population from Gran Canaria. *American Journal of Physical Anthropology* 128: 560-568.

De Soet, J.J. & Laine, M.L. (2008). Genetics and caries [Article in Dutch] Ned Tijdschr Tandheelkd 115 (2):78-82.

Donald, A.M. (2004) Understanding starch structure and functionality. In: Eliasson, A.C. (Ed.) *Starch in food. Structure, function and applications*. Woodhead Publishing Limited, Cambridge UK.

Donnelly, C.J., Thomson, L.A., Stiles, H.M., Brewer, C., Neel, J.V. & Brunelle, J.A. (1977). Plaque, caries, periodontal diseases and accumulations among Yanomano Indians, Venezuela. *Community Dentistry and Oral Epidemiology* 5(1): 30-39.

Dosi, A. & Schnell, F. (1990). *A tavala con i Romani Antichi*. Nuova Editrice Romana, Roma.

Dowd, F.J. (1999). Saliva and dental caries. *Dental Clinics of North America* 43:579–597.

Duyar, I. & Erdal, Y.S. (2003). A new approach for calibrating dental cáries frequency of skeletal remains. *Homo, Journal of Comparative Human Biology* 54: 57-70.

Esclassan, R., Grimoud, A.M., Ruas, M.P., Donat, R., Sevin, A., Astie, F., Lucas, S. & Crubezy, E. (2009). Dental caries, tooth wear and diet in an adult medieval (12th-14th century) population from mediterranean France. *Archives of Oral Biology* 54: 287–297.

Eshed, V.; Gopher, A. & Hershkovitz, I. (2006). Tooth wear and dental pathology at the advent of agriculture: new evidence from the Levant. *American Journal of Physical Anthropology* 130(2):145-59.

Fejerskov, O., Larsen, M.J., Richards, A. & Baelum, V. (1994). Dental Tissue Effects of Fluoride. *Advances in Dental Research* 8(1): 15-31.

Frayer, D.W. (1984). Tooth size, oral pathology and class distinctions: evidence from the Hungarian Middle Ages. *Anthropologiai Közlemenyek* 28, 47-54.

Frayer, D.W. (1976). *Evolutionary Dental Changes in Upper Paleolithic and Mesolithic Human Populations, vols. 1 and 2.* Ph. D. Thesis. University of Michigan. University Microfilms n° 76-19,136.

Frostell, G., Keyes, P.H. & Larson, A. (1967). Effect of various sugars and sugar substitutes on dental caries in hamsters and rats. *Journal of Nutrition* 93: 65-73.

Fry, B. (2006). *Stable isotope ecology.* Springer Science and Business Media LLC, New York.

Gagnon, C.M. (2004). Food and the state: Bioarchaeological investigations of diet in the Moche valley of Perú. *Dental Anthropology* 17 (2): 45-53.

Godoy, M.C. (2005). *Tiwanaku and Chiribya: Diet and dental diseases during the Middle Horizon and Late Intermediate Period in de Lower Osmore Valley.* M.Sc. Dissertation. University College London Institute of Archaeology, London.

Götze, W., Mengede, P. & Fulde, T. (1986). Periodontal and oral hygiene status and caries incidence in bakers and confectioners. *Zahnärztliche Welt, Zahnärztliche Rundshau* 95(1): 50-2.

Gorrel, C. (2006). *Odontología Veterinaria en la práctica clínica.* Ed. Servet, Zaragoza.

Grenby, T.H. (1997). Summary of the dental effects of starch. *International Journal of food sciences and nutrition* 48: 411-416.

Grine, F.E., Gwinnett, A.J. & Oaks, J.H. (1990). Early hominid dental pathology: Interproximal caries in 1.5 million-year-old *Paranthropus robustus* from Swartkrans. *Archives of Oral Biology* 35, 5: 381-386.

Gustafsson, B.E., Quensel, C.E., Swenander, L., Lundqvist, C., Grahnn, H., Bonow, E. & Krasse, B. (1953). The effect of different levels of carbohydrate intake on cáries activity in 436 individuals observed for five years. *Acta Odontologica Scandinavica* 11, 3 & 4: 232 – 364.

Harris, J.E., Iskander, Z. & Farid, S. (1975). Restorative dentistry in ancient Egypt: An archaeological fact. *Journal Michigan Dental Association* 57, 401-404.

Hassell, T.M. & Harris, E.L. (1995) Genetic influences in caries and periodontal diseases. *Critical Reviews in Oral Biology and Medicine* 6(4): 319-42.

Haugejorden, O. (1996). Using the DMF gender difference to assess the 'major' role of fluoride toothpastes in the caries decline in industrialized countries: a meta-analysis. *Community Dentistry and Oral Epidemiology* 24:369–375.

Heredia, C. & Alva, F. (2005). Relación entre la prevalencia de caries dental y desnutrición crónica en niños de 5 a 12 años de edad. *Revista Estomatológica Herediana* 15, 2: 124-127.

Hillson, S.W. (2001). Recording dental caries in archaeological human remains. *International Journal of Osteoarchaeology* 11: 249–289.

Hillson, S. (2008). Dental Pathology. In: *Biological Anthropology of the Human Skeleton.* Katzenberg, M.A. & Saunders, S.R. (Eds). pp. 249–286. Wiley-Liss, New York.

Hollister, M.C. & Weintraub, J.A. (1993). The association of oral status with systemic health, quality of life, and economic productivity. *Jounal of Dental Education* 57:901-912

Holloway, P.J., James, P.M.C. & Slack, G.L. (1963). Dental disease in Tristan da Cunha. *British Dental Journal* 115: 19–25.

Indriati, E. & Buikstra, J.E. (2001). Coca chewing in prehistoric coastal Peru: dental evidence. *American Journal of Physical Anthropology* 114:242-257.

Ismail, A.L., Tanzer, J.M. & Dingle, J.I. (1997). Current trends of sugar consumption in developing societies. *Community Dentistry and Oral Epidemiology* 25: 438-445.

Jackson, R. (1988). *Doctors and disease in the Roman Empire.* British Museum Publications, London.

Kainz, E. & Sonnabend, E. (1983). Evaluation of caries incidence in a pastry chefs' school. *Zahnärztliche Welt, Zahnärztliche Rundshau* 92(12): 60-2.

Katzenberg, A.M. & Saunders, S.R. (Eds.) (2008). Biological Anthropology of the Human Skeleton. 2nd edition. Willey-Liss, New Jersey.

Kear, B.P. (2001). Dental caries in an Early Cretaceous ichthyosaur. *Alcheringa: an Australian journal of palaeontology* 25(4): 387-390.

Kemp, A. (2003). Dental and skeletal pathology in lungfish jaws and tooth plates. *Alcheringa: an Australian journal of palaeontology* 27(2): 155-170.

Keene, H.J. (1986). Dental caries prevalence in early Polynesians from the Hawaiian Islands. *Journal of Dental Research* 65:935–938.

Keenleyside, A. (1998). Skeletal evidence of health and disease in pre-contact Alaskan Eskimos and Aleuts. *American Journal of Physical Anthropology* 107:51-70.

Kelley, M.A; Levesque, D.R. & Weidl, E. (1991). Contrasting patterns of dental disease in five early northern Chilean groups. In: *Advances in dental anthropology.* Kelley, M.A. & Larsen, C.S. (Eds.). pp. 203–213. Wiley-Liss, New York.

Kerr, N.W., Bruce, M.F. & Cross, J.F. (1990). Caries in Mediaeval Scots. *American Journal of Physical Anthropology* 83: 69–76.

Kilgore, L. (1989). Dental pathologies in ten free ranging chimpanzees from Gombe National Park, Tanzania. *American Journal of Physical Anthropology* 80: 219–237.

King, T., Humphrey, L.T. & Hillson, S. (2005). Linear enamel hypoplasias as indicators of systemic physiological stress: Evidence from two known age-at-death and sex populations from postmedieval London. *American Journal of Physical Anthropology* 128: 547–559.

Lalueza, C., Pérez-Pérez, A., Chimenos, E., Maroto, J. & Turbón, D. 1993. Estudi radiogràfic i mcroscòpic de la mandíbula de Banyoles: patologies i estat de conservación. In: Maroto, J. (Ed.), *La Mandíbula de Banyoles en el context dels fossils humans del Pleistocè. Sèrie Monogràfica,* vol. 13. pp. 135-144. Centre d'Investigacions Arqueològiques de Girona.

Langsjöen, O.M. (1996). Dental effects of diet and coca-leaf chewing on two prehistoric cultures of northern Chile. *American Journal of Physical Anthropology* 101: 475-489.

Larsen, C.S. (1997) *Bioarchaeology: Interpreting behavior from the human skeleton.* Cambridge University Press, New York.

Larsen, C.S., Shavit, R. & Griffin, M.C. (1991). Dental Caries Evidence for Dietary Change: An Archaeological Context. In: *Advances in dental anthropology.* Kelley, M.A. & Larsen, C.S. (Eds.). pp.179–202. Wiley-Liss, New York;

Lebel, S. & Trinkaus, E. (2001). A carious Neandertal molar from the Bau de l'Aubesier, Vaucluse, France. *Journal of Archaeological Science* 28:555-557.

Leung, F. (1981). Mills and Milling in Upper Canada. Ontario Government Publications, History and Archives 53, Ontario.

Lieverse, A.R., Weber, A.W., Bazaliiskiy, V.I., Goriunova, O.I. & Savelev, N.A. (2007). Dental health indicators of hunter–gatherer adaptation and cultural change in Siberia's Cis-Baikal. *American Journal of Physical Anthropology* 134:323–339.

Lingström, P. & Borrman, H. (1999). Distribution of dental caries in an Early 17th century Swedish population with special reference to diet. *International Journal of Osteoarchaeology* 9: 395–403.

Lingström, P.; Van Houte, J. & Kashket, S. (2000). Food, starches and dental caries. *Critical Reviews in Oral Biology and Medicine* 11(3): 366-380.

López, B., García-Vázquez, E. & Dopico, E. (2011). Dental Indicators Suggest Health Improvement Associated with Increased Food Diversity in Modern Age Spain. *Human Ecology*. Published on line 10 May 2011 - DOI 10.1007/s10745-011-9406-y.

Luan, W.M., Baelum, V., Chen, X. & Fejerskov, O. (1989). Dental caries in adult and elderly Chinese. *Journal of Dental Research* 68: 1771-1776.

Lubell, D., Jackes, M., Schwarcz, H., Knyf, M. & Meiklejohn, C. (1994). The Mesolithic-Neolithic transition in Portugal: isotopic and dental evidence of diet. *Journal of Archaeological Science* 21, 201-216.

Lukacs, J.R. (1990). On hunter gatherers and the neighbors in prehistoric India: contact and pathology. *Current Anthropology* 31, 183-6.

Lukacs, J.R. (1992). Dental paleopathology and agricultural intensification in South Asia: New evidence from Bronze Age Harappa. *American Journal of Physical Anthropology* 87: 133-50.

Lukacs, J.R. (1996). Sex differences in dental caries rates with the origin of Agriculture in South Asia. *Current Anthropology*, Vol. 37, No. 1: 147-153.

Lukacs, J.R. (2007). Dental trauma and antemortem tooth loss in prehistoric canary islanders: Prevalence and contributing factors. *International Journal of Osteoarchaeology* 17: 157–173.

Lukacs, J.R. (2008). Fertility and agriculture accentuate sex differences in dental caries rates. *Current Anthropology* 49, 5: 901-914.

Lukacs, J.R. (2011). Sex differences in dental caries experience: clinical evidence, complex etiology. *Clinical Oral Investigations* 15:649–656.

Lukacs, J.R. & Largaespada, L. (2006). Explaining sex differences in dental caries prevalence: saliva, hormones, and "life-history" aetiologies. *American Journal of Human Biology* 18(4):540-55.

Lull, V., González Marcén, P. & Risch, R. (1991). *Arqueología de Europa, 2250-1200 A.C.: Una introducción a la Edad del Bronce*. Editorial Síntesis, Madrid.

Maat, G.J.R. & Van der Velde, E.A. 1987. The caries-attrition competition. *International Journal of Anthropology* 2:281–292.

Manzi, G., Salvadei, L., Vienna, A. & Passarello, P. (1999). Discontinuity of life conditions at the transition from the Roman Imperial age to the Early Middle Ages: example from central Italy evaluated by pathological dento–alveolar lesions. *American Journal of Human Biology* 11: 327–341.

Martinón-Torres, M., Martín-Francés, L., Gracia, A., Olejniczak, A., Prado-Simón, L., Gómez-Robles, A., Lapresa, M., Carbonell, E., Arsuaga, J. & Bermúdez de Castro, J.M. (2011) Early Pleistocene human mandible from Sima del Elefante (TE) cave site in Sierra de Atapuerca (Spain): A palaeopathological study. *Journal of Human Evolution* 61: 1-11.

Matthesen, M., Baelum, V. & Aarslev, L. (1986). Dental health of children and adults in Guinea-Bissau, West Africa in 1986. *Community Dental Health* 7:123-33.

Mayhall, J.T. (1970). The effect of culture change upon the Eskimo dentition. *Arctic Anthropology* 7(1):117-121.

Mayhall, J.T. (1977). The oral health of a Canadian Inuit community: an anthropological approach. *Journal of Dental Research* 56: C55-61.

Mazzi, M.S. (1981). Consumi alimentari e malattie nel basso medioevo. *Archeologia medievale* 8: 321-336.

Medronho, R.A., Bloch, K.V., Luiz, R.R. & Werneck, G.L. (2009). *Epidemiologia*. 2a ed. Editora Atheneu. São Paulo.

Meiklejohn, C., Wyman, J.M. & Schentag, C.T. (1992). Caries and attrition: Dependent or independent variables? *International Journal of Anthropology* 7: 17-22.

Mellquist, C. & Sandberg, T. (1939). Odontological studies of about 1400 medieval skulls from Halland and Scania in Sweden and from Norse colony in Greenland and a contribution to the knowledge of their anthropology. *Odontologisk Tidskrift* 47: 2–83.

Miles, A. & Grigson, C. (1990). Other Disorders of Teeth and Jaws-Periodontal disease. In: *Colyer's Variations and Diseases of the Teeth of Animals. Revised Edition.* Miles, A., Grigson, C. (Eds.). pp.532-535.Cambridge University Press, Cambridge.

Milner, G.R. (1984). Dental caries in the permanent dentition of a Mississippian period population from the American Midwest. *Collegium Anthropologicum* 8: 77-91.

Milner, G.R. & Larsen, C.S. (1991). Teeth as artifacts of human behavior: intentional mutilation and accidental modification. In: *Advances in dental anthropology.* Kelley, M.A. & Larsen, C.S. (Eds.). pp. 357-378. Willey Liss, New York.

Molnar, S. (1972). Tooth wear and culture: A survey of tooth functions among some prehistoric populations. *Current Anthropology* 13: 511-526.

Moore, W.J. (1993). Dental caries in Britain. In: *Food, Diet and Economic Change Past and Present.* Geissler, C. & Oddy, D.J. (Eds.). pp. 50–61. Leicester University Press, Leicester.

Moore, W.J. & Corbett, M.E. (1971) The distribution of dental caries in ancient British populations. I. Anglo-Saxon period. *Caries Research* 5:151–168.

Moore, W.J. & Corbett, M.E. (1973) The distribution of dental caries in ancient British populations. II. Iron Age, Romano-British and Mediaeval periods. *Caries Research* 7:139-153.

Moore, W.J. & Corbett, M.E. (1975) Distribution of dental caries in ancient British populations. III. The 17th century. *Caries Research* 9:163-175.

Nelson, G.C. & Lukacs, J. R. (1994). Early antemortem tooth loss due to caries in a late Iron Age sample from the Sultanate of Oman. *American Iournal of Physical Anthropology* supp. 18:152.

Nelson, G.C., Lukacs, J. R. & Yule, P. (1999). Dates, caries, and early tooth loss during the Iron Age of Oman. *American Journal of Physical Anthropology* 108:333–343.

Neves, W.A. & Cornero, S. (1997). What did South American paleoinidans eat? *Current Research Pleistocene* 14, 93-96.

Nikiforouk, G. (1985) *Understanding dental caries.* Basel Karger, New York.

Nikiforouk, G., Fraser, D. (1981). The etiology of enamel hypoplasia: a unifying concept. *Journal of Pediatrics* 98: 888.

Ogilvie, M.D., Curran, B.K. & Trinkaus, E. (1989). Incidence and patterning of dental enamel hypoplasia among the Neandertals. *American Journal of Physical Anthropology* 79(1):25-41.

Okumura, M. & Eggers, S. (2005). The people of Jabuticabeira II: Reconstruction of the way of life in a Brazilian shellmound. *Homo, Journal of Comparative Human Biology* 55: 263-281.

Osborn, T.W. & Noriskin, J.N. (1937). The Relation Between Diet and Caries in the South African Bantu. *Journal of Dental Research* (16): 431-441.

Palamra, J., Phakey, P.P., Rachinger, W.A. & Orams, H.J. (1981). The Ultrastructure of Enamel from the Kangaroo Macropus giganteus: Tubular Enamel and its 'Black Spots' Defect. *Australian Journal of Zoology* 29 (4): 643-652.

Pando, R. (1988). *Estudio comparativo de prevalencia de caries, enfermedad periodontal y abrasión entre un grupo de sujetos con el hábito de masticar hojas de coca y un grupo control en la comunidad de Punray*. Provincia de Tarma, Departamento de Junín. Bachelor Thesis. Universidad Peruana Cayetano Heredia, Lima.

Parker, M. (2011). *The Sugar Barons: Family, Corruption, Empire and War*. Hutchinson, London.

Pearsall, D. (2000). *Paleoethnobotany: A handbook of procedures*. Second edition. Academic Press, California.

Pechenkina, E.A., Benfer Jr., R.A. & Zhijun, W. (2002). Diet and health changes at the end of the Chinese Neolithic: The Yangshao/Longshan transition in Shaanxi province. *American Journal of Physical Anthropology* 117:15-36.

Pedersen, P.O. (1947). Dental investigations of Greenland Eskimos. *Proceedings of the Royal Society of Medicine* 40:726-732.

Pedersen, P.O. (1952). Some dental aspects of anthropology. *Dental Record* 72:170-178.

Pedersen, P.O. (1971). Dental caries in Greenland 1935-1969. Pre-war Greenland and its population. *DtschZahnarztl-Z.* 26:1023.

Petersen, P.E. & Razanamihaja, N. (1996). Oral health status of children and adults in Madagascar. *International Dental Journal* 46:41–47.

Petersen, P.E. & Kaka M. (1999). Oral health status of children and adults in the Republic of Niger, Africa. *International Dental Journal* 49:159–64.

Pérez Samper, M.A. (2003). La alimentación en la corte española del siglo XVIII. *Cuadernos de Historia Moderna* Anejo II, 153-197.

Pezo-Lanfranco, L. (2010). *Reconstrução de padres paleopatológicos dentais em agricultores incipientes e desenvolvidos do litoral dos Andes Centrais*. M.Sc. Dissertation. Instituto de Biociências. Universidade de São Paulo. São Paulo.

Pezo-Lanfranco, L. & Eggers, S. (2010). The usefulness of caries frequency, depth and location in determining cariogenicity and past subsistence: a test on early and later agriculturalists from the Peruvian coast. *American Journal of Physical Anthropology* 143:75–91.

Pinto, A.C. & Etxebarria, F. (2001). Patologías óseas en un esqueleto de Oso pardo macho adulto de la Cordillera Cantábrica (Reserva Nacional de Caza de Riaño, León). *Cadernos Lab. Xeolóxico de Laxe.* 26: 564-477.

Piperno, D. (2011). Northern Peruvian Early and Middle Preceramic Agriculture in Central and South American Contexts. In: *From Foraging to Farming in the Andes. New Perspectives on Food Production and Social Organization*. Dillehay, T. (Ed.). pp. 274-284. Cambridge University Press, New York.

Powell, M.L. (1985). The analysis of dental wear and caries for dietary reconstruction. In: Gilbert, R.I. & Mielke, L.J.H. (Eds.). *The analysis of prehistoric diets*. pp. 307–338. Academic Press, New York.

Powell, M.L. (1988). *Status and health in prehistory: A case study of the Moundville chiefdom.* Smithsonian Institution Press, Washington DC.

Prats, J. & Rey, C. (2003) *Las bases modernas de la alimentación tradicional.* Instituto de Estudios Almerienses. Available from: http://dialnet.unirioja.es/servlet/oaiart?codigo=2246686.

Puech, P.F.F. (1995). Dentistry in ancient Egypt: Junkers' teeth. *Dental anthropology newsletter* 10(1): 5-7.

Reed, DM. (1994) Ancient Maya diet at Copan, Honduras, as determined through isotopes. In: *Paleonutrition: the diet and health of prehistoric Americans.* Sobolik, K.D. (Ed.). pp. 210-21. Center of Archaeological Investigation, occasional paper, 22. University of Carbondale, Southern Illinois.

Roberts, C.M. & Manchester, K. (Eds.). (2005). *The archaeology of disease.* 3rd edition. Cornell University Press, New York.

Robinson, J.T. (1952). Some hominid features of the ape-man dentition. *Journal Dent Association of South Africa* 7: 102-113.

Rodríguez, JV. (2003) *Dientes y diversidad humana, Avances de la antropología dental.* Editorial Guadalupe Ltda, Bogotá.

Rugg-Gunn, A.J. & Edgar, W.M. (1984) Sugar and dental caries: A review of the evidence. *Community Dental Health* I:85-92.

Rugg-Gunn, A.J. & Hackett, A.F. (1993). *Nutrition and dental health.* Oxford University Press, New York.

Sakashita, R., Inoue, M., Inoue, N., Pan Q. & Zhu, H. (1997). Dental disease in the chinese Yin-Shang period with respect to relationships between citizens and slaves. *American Journal Physical Anthropology* 103:401-408.

Saunders, S., De Vito, C. & Katzenberg, A. (1997). Dental caries in nineteenth century Upper Canada. *American Journal of Physical Anthropology* 104:71-87.

Sala, N., Cuevas, J. & López, N. (2007). Estudio paleopatológico de una hemimandíbula de Tethytragus (Artiodactyla, Mammalia) del Mioceno Medio de Somosaguas (Pozuelo de Alarcón, Madrid). *Colóquios de Paleontología* 57: 7-14.

Salvolini, E., Di Giorgio, R., Curatola, A., Mazzanti, L. & Fratto, G. (1998). Biochemical modifications of human whole saliva induced by pregnancy. *British Journal of Obstetrics and Gynaecology* 195:656-660.

Schamschula, H.G., Cooper, M.H., Wright, H.C. & Agus, H.M. (1980). Oral health of adolescent and adult Australian aborigines. *Community Dentistry and Oral Epidemiology* 8(7): 370-374.

Schultz, A.H. (1956). The occurrence and frequency of pathological and teratological conditions and of twinning among non-human primates. In: *Primatologia-Handbook of Primatology Vol 1.* Hofer, H., Schultz, A.H. & Starck, D. (Eds.). pp. 965-101. Karger Basel, New York.

Shafer, W.G., Hine, M.K. & Levy, B.W. (1983). *A textbook of oral pathology.* 4th ed. Saunders, Philadelphia.

Sharpe, P. (1998). *Sugar Cane: Past and Present.* Southern Illinois University, Illinois.

Shuler, C.F. (2001). Inherited risks for susceptibility to dental caries. *Journal of Dentistry Education* 65 (10): 1038-45.

Shaw, J.H. (1985). Diet and dental health. *American Journal of Clinical Nutrition* 41:1117-1131.

Shklair, I.L. (1981) Natural occurence of caries in animals. Animals as vector and reservoirs of cariogenic flors. In: Tanzer, J.M. (Ed.). *Animal Models in Cariology.* pp. 41-8. Information Retrieval, Washington.

Šlaus, M., Bedic, Z., Rajic, P., Vodanovic, M. & Kunic, A., (2011). Dental Health at the Transition from the Late Antique to the Early Medieval Period on Croatia's Eastern Adriatic Coast. *International Journal of Osteoarchaeology* 21: 577–590.

Swärstedt, T. (1966). *Odontological aspects of a medieval population in the province of Jämtland/Mid Sweden.* Tiden-Barnängen Tryckerier, Stockolm.

Tayles, N., Dommet, K. & Nelsen, K. (2000). Agriculture and dental cáries? The case of rice in prehistoric Southeast Asia. *World Archaeology* 32(1): 68–83.

Tayles, N., Domett, K, & Halcrow, S. (2009). Can dental caries be interpreted as evidence of farming? The Asian experience. *Frontiers of Oral Biology* 13: 162-166.

Taylor, R.E. (1987). *Radiocarbon dating: An archaeological perspective.* Academic Press, Orlando.

Teschler-Nichola, M., Knissel, M., Brandstätter, F. & Prossinger, H. (1998). A recently discovered Etruscan dental bridgework. In: *Dental Anthropology. Fundamentals, Limits, and Prospects.* Alt, K.W., Rösing, F.W. & Teschler-Nicola M. (Eds.). pp. 57-68. Springer, Wien, New York.

Tillier, A.M., Arensburg, B., Rak, Y. & Vandermeersch, B., (1995). Middle Palaeolithic dental caries: new evidence from Kebara (Mount Carmen, Israel). *Journal of Human Evolution* 29: 189-192.

Touger-Decker, R. & Loveren, C. (2003). Sugars and dental caries. *Nutrition* 78 (supl.): 8815-8925.

Trinkaus, E., Smith, R. & Lebel, S. (2000). Dental Caries in the Aubesier 5 Neandertal Primary Molar. *Journal of Archaeological Science* 27: 1017–1021. doi: 10.1006/jasc.1999.0512

Turner, C. (1978). Dental caries and early Ecuadorian agriculture. *American Antiquity* 43 (4): 694-697.

Turner, C. (1979). Dental anthropological indications of agriculture among the Jomon people of central Japan. *American Journal Physical Anthropology* 51:619–636.

Ubelaker, D.H. (2000) Human Remains from La Florida, Quito, Ecuador. *Smithsonian Contributions to Anthropology, n° 43.* Smithsonian Institution Press, Washington DC.

Ungar, P.S., Grine, F.E., Teaford, M. & Pérez-Pérez, A. (2001) A review of interproximal wear grooves on fossil hominid teeth with new evidence from Olduvai Gorge. *Archives of Oral Biology* 46: 285-292.

Valdéz, I.H., Atkinson, J.C. & Ship, J.A. (1993). Major salivary gland function in patients with radiation-induced xerostomia: flow rates and sialochemistry. International Journal of Radiat Oncology Biology Physiology 25:41-47.

Valdivia, L. (1980). *Odonto-antropología peruana.* Consejo Nacional de Ciencia y Tecnología CONCYTEC. Lima.

van Palenstein, W., Matee, M., van der Hoeven, J. & Mikx, F. (1996). Cariogenicity Depends More on Diet than the Prevailing Mutans Streptococcal Specie. *Journal of dental Research* 75 (1): 535-545.

Varrela, T.M. (1991). Prevalence and distribution of dental caries in a late medieval population in Finland. *Archives of Oral Biology* 36: 553-559.

Vodanovic, M., Brkic, H., Slaus, M. & Demo, Z. (2005). The frequency and distribution of caries in the mediaeval population of Bijelo Brdo in Croatia (10th—11th century). *Archives of Oral Biology* 50, 669—680.

Waldron, T. (2009). *Palaeopathology. Cambridge Manuals in Archaeology.* Cambridge University Press, New York.

Walker, P.L. & Erlandson, J.M. (1986). Dental evidence for prehistoric dietary change on the northern Channel Islands, California. *American Antiquity* 51(2):375-383.

Walker, P.L. & Hewlett, B.S. (1990). Dental health, diet and social status among central African foragers and farmers. *American Anthropologist* 92: 382-98.

Walker, M..J., Zapata, J., Lombardi, A.V. & Trinkaus, E. (2011). New Evidence of Dental Pathology in 40,000-year-old Neandertals. *Journal of Dental Research* 90 (4): 428-432.

Watt, M.E., Lunt, D.A. & Gilmouv, B.H. (1997). Caries prevalence in the permanent dentition of a mediaeval population from the southwest of Scotland. *Archives of Oral Biology* 42 (9): 601-620.

Wesolowski, V. (2006). Caries prevalence in skeletal series – Is it possible to compare? *Memoria do Instituto Oswaldo Cruz, Rio de Janeiro* 101 (Supll. II):139-145.

White, C.D. (1994). Dietary Dental Pathology and Cultural Change in the Maya. In: *Strength in Diversity.* Herring, D.A. & Chan, L. (Eds.). pp. 279–302. Canadian Scholar's Press, Toronto.

Wiggs, R. & Lobprise, H. (1997). *Veterinary dentistry: principles and practice.* Lippincott-Raven Publishers, Philadelphia.

Wrangham, R. (2009). *Catching fire: How cooking made us human.* Basic Books, New York.

2

Impacted Teeth and Their Influence on the Caries Lesion Development

Amila Brkić

Sarajevo University, School of Dental Medicine,
Department of Oral Surgery and Dental Implantology, Sarajevo,
Bosnia and Herzegovina

1. Introduction

In oral and maxillofacial surgery removal of impacted teeth, especially third molars is one of the most performed surgical procedures. Several studies suggest that a millions of dollars are spend annually on the management of the impacted teeth (Edwards et al.,1999; Flick, 1999).

By definition, impacted or unerupted tooth is one that lying within the jaws and fails to erupt into the dental arch with the expected time (Jojić & Perović, 1990; Hupp et al. 2008). Detected clinically and radiographically, there are two types of impactions; completely and partially. Completely impaction means that the tooth is prevented from completely erupting into a normal functional position, covered by bone and mucosa, while partially impaction implies that the tooth is partially visible or in communication with oral cavity, but it has failed to erupt fully into a normal position (Jojić & Perović, 1990).

Any permanent tooth can become impacted (Gisakis et al.,2010). Impaction is an abnormality of development which predisposes to pathological changes and complications such as pericoronitis and /or orofacial infection, periodontitis, root resorption of adjacent teeth, caries, odontogenic cysts and tumors. Also orthodontic and prothetic problems including temporomandibular joint (TMJ) symptomes should not be neglected (Knutsson et al., 1996; Punwutikorn et al., 1999). Because of the mentioned, many authors to prevent these complications suggest so called „early or prophilactic removal of impacted teeth", although in cases of patients who are free of symptoms or associated, this necessity is under the question (Gisakis et al.,2010). Patients between 20 and 30 years of age are the most frequently affected with symptomatic impactions (Sasano et al.,2003; Knutsson et al. 1996). As age increases, the phenomen of impaction is reduced and after the age of 50 it is at range from 6-14% (Ahlqwist & Grondahl, 1991; Gisakis et al.,2010).

From the last 40 years, an incidence of impacted teeth is growing through different populations, due to living habits such as feading by a „soft food" and lower intensity of the use of the masticatory aparatus (Alling et al., 1993). Only a few decades earlier, Inuits and Latin American Indians through feading habits were described as the populations with no impacted teeth (Jojic & Perović, 1990). Also, some authors suggest that race and gender have an influence on occurrence of impactions, thus the impactions are more common in Whites than Blacks (Brown et al., 1982), and females are more predisposed to this phenomenon than males (Jojic & Perović, 1990). However, by Haidar and Schalhoub (1986) in Saudi population, especially in cases of impacted third molars, male are more prone to have an impacted teeth than female patients.

2. Impacted teeth

The reasons for tooth impaction might include a several factors such as position and size of adjacent teeth, dense overlying bone, excessive soft tissue or a genetic abnormality including abnormal eruption path, dental arch length and space in which to erupt (Jojic & Perović, 1990; Alling et al., 1993; Hupp et al., 2008). Generally speaking these factors are subdivided into a two groups as local and general factors. The most common impacted teeth are mandibular and maxillary third molars, followed by the maxillary canines and mandibular premolars (Jojic & Perović, 1990; Hupp et al., 2008). Third molars have inadequate space for eruption, thus they are the last teeth to erupt. New data suggests that 72,7% of the world population has at least one impacted tooth (usually lower third molar), and it is more frequently in female than the male patients (Ahlqwist & Grondahl, 1991; Alling et al., 1993,).

Although indications for removal of impacted teeth vary from orthodontics, prosthodontics, pathologic and prophylactic, one of the reasons that impacted teeth should be removed, is their influence on the adjacent teeth with development of the caries lesions.

Caries is mentioned as one of the common pathological features associated with extracted mandibular third molars (Battaineh et al.,2002; Lysell & Rohlin, 1988; Punwutikom et al., 1999). This is a reason why in this section the emphasis will be on these teeth.

There is an opinion that the tooth position and inclination play a main roles in caries development process (Knutsson et al.,1996). For better understanding this relationship it is necessary to know a classification of impacted lower third molars. The most common used classification is by Winter in which third molars are classificated by their long axis angulation with respect to the long axis of adjacent second molars. Mesioangular position is the most seen type of third molar impaction comprising 43% of all third molar impactions, characterized by mesial direction of the third molar's long axis toward to the second molar with convergency angle of >30 (Kan et al., 2002). In vertical position, the long axis of impacted tooth runs parallel to the long axis of the second molar comprising 38%. Distoangular position including 6% of the cases is characterized by distally or posteriorly angled long axis of the tooth away from the second molar. If the long axis of the impacted tooth is perpendicular to the second molar comprising 3% of all cases, this position is known as the horizontal (Kan et al., 2002; Hupp et al., 2008). However, atypic positions in which impacted teeth are angled in buccal, linqual, palatal or buccolinqual directions are also recorded (Jojic & Perović, 1990; Hupp et al,. 2008). .

The second also in use classification is by Pell and Gregory, in which are described three positions of the third molars: depending of the relation of tooth to ramus and second molar subtypes (Type A), relative depth of the third molar in bone (Type B) tooth on same level with occlusal plane and position of long axis of the impacted tooth in relation to the second molar as taken from the Winter classification (Type C). (Kan et al., 2002; Hupp et al., 2008).

The practice suggests that horizontal and mesioangular positions are more critical to adjacent second molar, because impacted teeth in these positions may impige and resorb a distal surface and root of the second molars (Knutsson et al.,1996).

2.1 Winter classification of impacted lower third molars

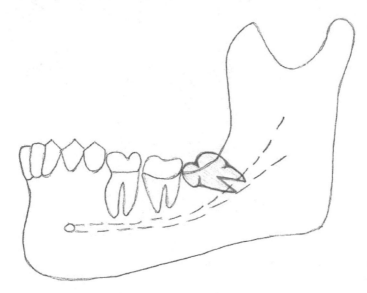

Fig. 1. Mesioangular position of the lower third molar.

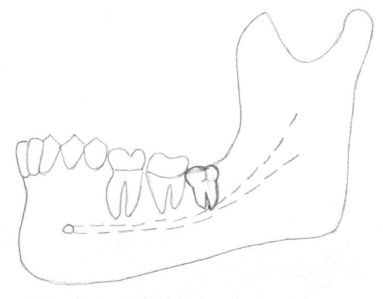

Fig. 2. Lower third molar in vertical position.

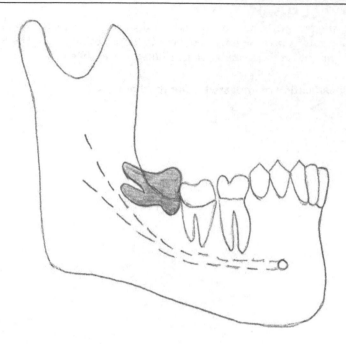

Fig. 3. Horizontal position of lower third molar.

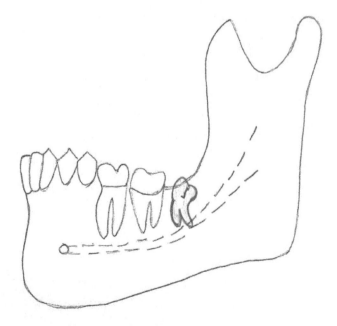

Fig. 4. Distoangular position of lower third molar.

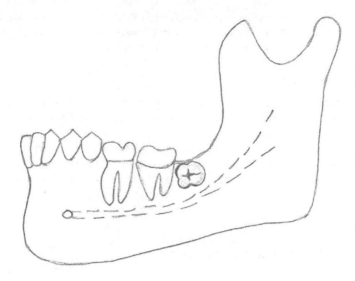

Fig. 5. Atipic position of the impacted tooth.

3. Caries

The most common causes of the tooth lost are caries and periodontal disease, following a tooth fracture (Jacobsen, 2008). Data suggests that in most industrialized countries 60-90 % of school aged children and almost 100% of adult population are affected by tooth decay (Petersen et al., 2005), with the prevalence, which is more higher in female than male (Lukacs & Largaespada, 2006; Ferraro & Vieira, 2010).

Tooth decay or dental caries is defined as chronic, multifactoral disease characterised by localized destruction of hard tooth tissues. It attacks on the mineralized tissues resulting in demineralization and in some cases destruction of the matrix (Jacobsen, 2008) . By some authors dental caries starts as small subclinical demineralised subsurface, which following a periods of remineralization and demineralization, may progress or arrest (Walmsley et al., 2002). There is an opinion that approximatelly 50 different factors subdivided into a three groups are in correlation with caries etiology: The first group is formed of those factors associated with the host such as quality of saliva and bacterial flora (Streptococcus mutans, Streptococcus sanquis, Actinomyces and Lactobacillae are the most commonly isolated from the caries lesions. These microorganisms produce lactic acid, also known as the milk acid, responsible for the caries development). The second group includes outside factors such as diet and the substrate on which bacteria act, while the third group content a tooth itself and those features which either predispose to or resist carious attack (Jacobsen, 2008).

Caries can affect enamel, dentin and cement, with usually localization at the cemento-enamel junction or in the cementum. However, in modern men grooves and fissure areas of the posterior teeth are the most common sites of decay (Newbrun,1989; Fejerskov & Kidd, 2008). There is a relationship between debth of the fissures and caries susceptibility, due to fact that food debris and microorganisms impact in the fissures. This leads to conclusion that a tooth morphology is an important determinant for the caries development. Due to gingival recesions and loss of periodontal and bone support, the root of the tooth may be exposed to the mouth and caries may occur (Jacobsen, 2008).

3.1 Impacted tooth - Caries

During tooth eruption into the oral cavity, organic pellicle and cellular covering which protect an enamel surface, are disepearing and on this way open the gate to attach of the saliva and microorganisms to the enamel (Jacobsen, 2008). In cases of impacted teeth, partially exposed impactions are the most prone to develop caries. Partially erupted tooth does not participate in mastication and for this reason offer more favorable conditions for bacterial accumulation than fully erupted tooth.(Fejerskov & Kidd, 2008) Due to fact that lower and upper third molars are the most common enclosed teeth, pericoronitis associated with bad oral hygiene and lesser self clening area, leads to food and microorganisam accumulation that can not be cleaned through normal brushings and flossing, causing a caries development. The crowns of mesio-angulary and horizontaly impacted third molars often interfares with registering pocket debth (Lenug et al., 2005) . Gingival swelling and inflammation may lead to the impression that the lesion is hiden in the pocket (Fejerskov & Kidd, 2008; Jacobsen, 2008). It is interesting that even under the gums and situations in which no obvious communication between the mouth and impacted tooth exist, tooth decay might be developed. In cases of partially impacted teeth occlusal and approximal sides are the most commonly affected. In extremly cases, a tooth crown might be completelly destroyed by the lesion.

For mesio-angular and horizontal impacted lower third molars partially exposed in the oral cavity, occlusal surfaces form plaque accumulative crevices against the distal surfaces of the second molars (Chu et al., 2003). On this way they cause a distal cervical caries on the second molars, though estimates of the rate vary from 1% to 4.5%, which is difficult to be restored without extractions of the impacted teeth. Also, as the gingival margin recedes enamel-cementum junction becomes exposed forming forming a bacterial retention side and on this way forming root surface caries (Jacobsen, 2008). McArdle & Rentol.(2006) suggests that second molar caries indication is responsible for 5% of mandibular third molar teeth removals. However, data from different authors suggests that these numbers are higher. Thus, van der Linden et al. (1995) reported caries in 7.1% of impacted third molars and in 42.7% of adjacent molars (204 and 1227 of 2872 teeth respectively). In study of Adeyemo et al.(2008) caries and its sequela (63,2%) was the major reason for the third molars extraction, followed by reccurent pericoronitis (26,3%) and periodontitis (9,2%). However in the study of Obiechina et al. (2001), pericoronitis and periodontal disease (42,92%) were the major reasons for the third molar removals. The incidence of the caries was 13,95%, and it was on the third place of the third molar teeth removal indications (Obiechina et al.,2001). Lysell & Rohlin (1998) showed that caries was associated with impacted third molars and second molars in 13% and 5% of cases respectively, Sasano et al.(2003) noted that 14.5% of symptomatic impactions were associated with dental caries. The results of Bataineh et al. (2002) showed an overall caries rate of 23% in impacted molars and 0.5% in the second molars associated with impacted molars. Knutsson et al. (1996) reported a high caries frequency of 31% with impactions, which was more common in patients between 20 and 29 years, followed by the 30 to 39 year group. Gisakis et al. (2011) reported an incidence of caries of the impacted and / or adjacent teeth of 9,9%. Allen et al. (2009) reported an incidence of 42% of the distal second molar caries associated with partially or completelly impacted third molars. By the same study distal angulation and the other types of inclinations were not associated with detectable caries (Allen et al.,2009) Chu et al. (2003) reported a caries rates in 2-3% of lower wisdom teeth , followed by 7,3% of the adjacent second molars. Because of the mentioned, some authors suggested that the early or prophylactic removal of a partially erupted mesioangular wisdom teeth could prevent distal cervical caries forming in the mandibular second molars (McArdle & Renton, 2006).

Caries lesions of partially impacted or adjacent teeth may or may not be cavitated, which is very important due to the fact that in cavitated lesions biofilms are more difficult to be controled by oral hygiene procedures. Cavitated lesions are the result of „undisturbed" dental plaque. In some cases tooth decay in the form of so called „hiden caries" might be present. This caries is characterized by lesion in demineralized dentin which is missed on a visual examination, but is detected radiographically (Newbrun, 1989). Radiographically, the caries lesion is in form of radiolucent zone, due to the fact that demineralized hard teeth tissues such as enamel and dentin do not absorbe a X-rays (Newbrun, 1989). Some dental practitioners in the cases of the asymptomatic partially impacted lower third molars in the vertical positions with caries lesion development, performe conservative therapy as repair of the cavity with placeing a filling. However, for this approach, to avoid a risk for development of the recurrent caries, an appropriate indication is necessary. This means that the patient's good oral hygiene without presence of dental plaque must be present.

In extreme cases, the tooth decay might be developed with great extension on the partially impacted third molars and adjacent second molars, that could not repeared with final result of the both teeth extractions (Walmsley et al., 2002).

Comparing with lower third molars, upper wisdom teeth are not often seen as the causer of the adjacent teeth distal caries.

Excluding a third molars, other impacted teeth may be also associated with caries risk. However, these findings are not so often seen.

Impacted upper canine is mostly in correlation with a rooth resorptions of the neighboring teeth, caries lesions of second incisor and the first premolar are not often seen in cases of the partially impacted canines. A position and inclination of supernumerary teeth, a product of hiperactivity of the dental lamina, also have an influence on the caries lesion developments. Meziodens as the clinically the most common supernumerary tooth, responsible for diastema of the central incisors, depending of localization, may cause a palatinal cervical and mesial caries lesions of the central incisors. Distomolar a supernumerary tooth located distal of the third molar, although it is rarely seen, might cause a distal caries of the neighbouring tooth.

4. Conclusion

Partially impaction of third molars play an important role in caries development of adjacent teeth. Mesio angular and horizontal positions are responsible for development of the distal cervical caries on the second molars, which is difficult to be restore without an extraction of impacted teeth. Early or prophilactic removal of a partially erupted mesio-angular and horizontal third molars could prevent distal cervical caries forming in the mandibular second molar. However, if the second molar has caries or large restoration, or has been endodonticaly treated, removal of partially or completelly impacted wisdom teeth, must to be safely performed without injuring the second molar. As one of the complications, it is expectable to be fracture restoration or a portion of the carious crown.

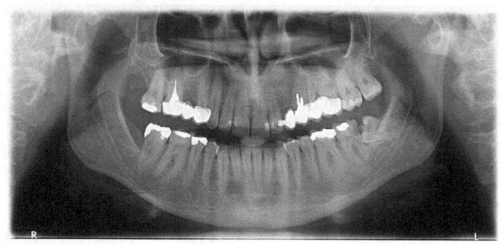

Fig. 6A. Partially impacted lower left wisdom tooth in horizontal position associated with the caries lesion on distal surface of the second molar.

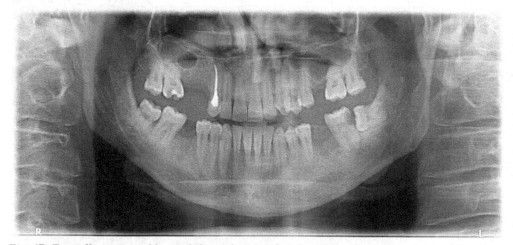

Fig. 6B. Partially impacted lower left wisdom tooth in horizontal position associated with the caries lesion on distal surface of the second molar.

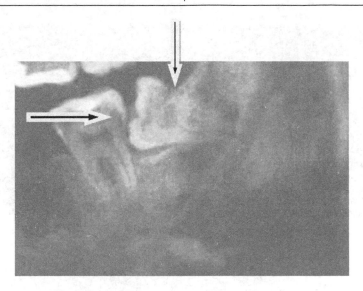

Fig. 7. The arrows show caries development on the distal surfaces of lower partially impacted third and second molar.

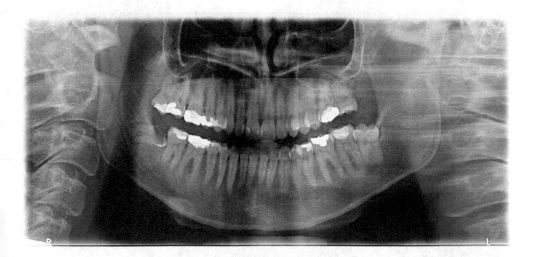

Fig. 8. Completelly destroyed by tooth decay, a crown of impacted lower right third molar tooth

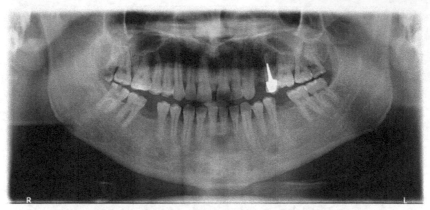

Fig. 9. Completelly destroyed by tooth decay, a crown of upper right third molar tooth.

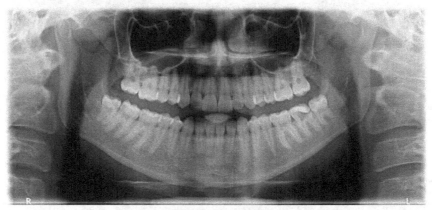

Fig. 10. Inadequate restoration of lower left second molar.

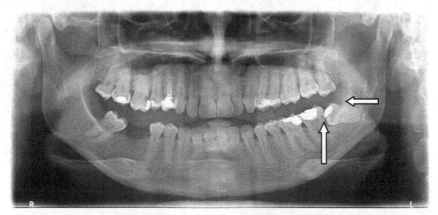

Fig. 11. Inadequate restoration of the oclusal surface of the lower left third molar. Arrows show a caries lesion beyond the filling and hiden caries of the distal surface of the second molar.

5. Acknowledgment

The author thanks Mr. Enes Tuna for technical support of the manuscript preparation.

6. References

Adeyemo, W.L., James, O., Ogunlewe, M.O., Ladeinde, A.L., Taiwo, O.A. & Olojede, A.C.(2008). Indications for extraction of third molars: a review of 1763 cases. *Niger Postgrad Med J.* Vol 15, No 1.pp. 42-46.

Ahlqwist, M. & Gröndahl, H.G.(1991). Prevalence of impacted teeth and associated pathology in middle-aged and older Swedish women. *Community Dent Oral Epidemiol.* Vol 19, No 2. pp. 116-119.

Akadiri, O.A., Okoje, V.N., Fasola, A.O., Olusanya, A.A. & Aladelusi, T.O.(2007). Indications for the removal of impacted mandible third molars at Ibadan--any compliance with established guidelines? *Afr J Med Med Sci.* Vol 36, No 4. pp.359-363.

Allen, R.T., Witherow, H., Collyer, J., Roper-Hall, R., Nazir, M.A. & Mathew, G.(2009). The mesioangular third molar--to extract or not to extract? Analysis of 776 consecutive third molars. *Br Dent J.* Vol 206, No 11. pp. 586-587.

Alling C.C, Helfrick J.F & Alling R.D. (1993). *Impacted Teeth.* W.B. Saunders. Philadelphia.

Bataineh, A.B., Albashaireh, Z.S. & Hazza'a, A.M.(2002). The surgical removal of mandibular third molars: a study in decision making. *Quintessence Int.* Vol 33, No 8. pp. 613-617.

Chu, F.C, Li, T.K., Lui, V.K., Newsome, P.R., Chow, R.L. & Cheung, L.K.(2003). Prevalence of impacted teeth and associated pathologies--a radiographic study of the Hong Kong Chinese population. *Hong Kong Med J.* Vol 9, No 3. pp.158-163. Edwards, M.J., Brickley,M.R., Goodey R.D.& Shepherd J.P.(1999). The cost, effectiveness and cost effectiveness of removal and retention of asymptomatic disease free third molars. *British Dental Journal.* Vol 187, No 7. pp. 38-44.

Fejerskov, O. & Kidd, E.(2008). *Dental caries. The disease and its clinical management* (2 nd edition), Blackwell Publishing Ltd, Oxford.

Ferraro, M. & Vieira, A. R.(2010). Explaining gender differences in caries: a multifactorial approach to a multifactorial disease. *Int J Dent.* 2010:649643. Epub 2010 Mar 16.

Flick, M.G.(1999). Third molar controversy: framing the controversy as a public health policy issue. *Journal of Oral and Maxillofacial surgery.* Vol. 57, No 4. pp. 438-444.

Gisakis, I.G, Palamidakis, F.D., Farmakis E.T.R, Kamberos, G. & Kamberos, S.(2011). Prevalence of impacted teeth in a Greek population. *Journal of Investigative and Clinical Dentistry* Vol 2, No2. pp.102–109.

Haidar, Z. & Shalhoub, S.Y.(1986). The incidence of impacted wisdom teeth in a Saudi community. *Int J Oral Maxillofac Surg.* Vol 15, No 5. pp. 569-571.

Hupp, J.R, Ellis III, E. & Tucker, M.R.(2008) *Contemporary oral and maxillofacial surgery* (5th edition), Mosby Elsevier, St. Louis, Missouri.

Jacobsen P.(2005). *Restorative dentistry. An integrated approach* (2nd edition), Blackwell Publishing Ltd, Singapore.

Jojić, B. & Perović, J.V.(1990). *Oralna hirurgija* (4th edition), Naučna knjiga, Beograd.

Kan, K. W., Liu, J. K. S., Lo, E. C. M., Corbet,E. F. & Leung, W. K. (2002) Residual periodontal defects distal to the mandibular second molar 6–36 months after impacted third molar extraction. *Journal of Clinical Periodontology* Vol 29, No 11. pp. 1004–1011.

Knutsson, K., Brehmer, B., Lysell, L. & Rohlin, M. (1996). Pathoses associated with mandibular third molars subjected to removal. *Oral Surg Oral Med Oral Pathol Oral Radiol and Endod*. Vol 82, No 1. pp.10-7.

Leung, W.K., Corbet, E.F., Kan, K.W., Lo, E.C. & Liu, J.K. (2005) A regimen of systematic periodontal care after removal of impacted mandibular third molars manages periodontal pockets associated with the mandibular second molars. *J Clin Periodontol*. Vol 32, No 7. pp. 725-731.

Lukacs, J. R. & Largaespada,L.L. (2006). Explaining sex differences in dental caries prevalence: saliva, hormones, and "life history" etiologies. *American Journal of Human Biology*, Vol. 18, No 4. pp. 540–555.

Lysell, L. & Rohlin, M.(1998). A study of indications used for removal of the mandibular third molar. *Int J Oral Maxillofac Surg*. Vol 17, No 3. pp.161-164.

McArdle, L.W. & Renton, T.F.(2006). Distal cervical caries in the mandibular second molar: an indication for the prophylactic removal of the third molar? *Br J Oral Maxillofac Surg*. Vol 44, No 1. pp. 42-45.

Newbrun, E (1989) *Cariology* (3rd edition), Quintessence publishing CO, Inc Chicago Illinois.

Obiechina, A. E., Arotiba, J.T. & Fasola, A.O.(2001). Third molar impaction: evaluation of the symptoms and pattern of impaction of mandibular third molar teeth in Nigerians. *Odontostomatol Trop*. Vol 24, No 93. pp.22-25.

Petersen, P.E., Bourgeois, D., Ogawa, H., Estupinan-Day, S & Ndiaye, C. (2005). The global burden of oral diseases and risks to oral health. *Bulletin of the World Health Organization*. Vol 83, No 9. pp. 661–669.

Polat, H.B, Ozan, F., Kara, I., Ozdemir, H.& Ay, S. (2008). Prevalence of commonly found pathoses associated with mandibular impacted third molars based on panoramic radiographs in Turkish population. *Oral Surg Oral Med Oral Pathol Oral Radiol Endod*. Vol 105, No 6. pp. e41-47.

Punwutikorn, J., Waikakul, A. & Ochareon, P.(1999). Symptoms of unerupted mandibular third molars. *Oral Surg Oral Med Oral Pathol Oral Radiol Endod*. Vol 87, No 3. pp.305-310.

Sasano, T., Kuribara, N., Iikubo, M., Yoshida A, et al. (2003). Influence of an angular position and degree of impaction of third molars on development of symptoms: Long term follow-up under good oral hygiene condition. *Tohoku Journal of Experimental Medicine*. Vol 200, No 2. pp.75-83.

Van der Linden, W., Cleaton-Jones, P. & Lownie, M.(1995). Diseases and lesions associated with third molars. Review of 1001 cases. *Oral Surg Oral Med Oral Pathol Oral Radiol Endod*. Vol 79, No 2. pp. 142-145.

Walmsley, A.D, Walsh, T.F., Trevor Burke, F.J., Shortall, A.C.C., Lumley, P.J. & Hayes – Hall, R. (2002). *Restorative dentistry*. Churcil Livingstone. Edinburgh.

3

Socioeconomic Influence on Caries Susceptibility in Juvenile Individuals with Limited Dental Care: Example from an Early Middle Age Population (Great Moravia, 9th-10th Centuries A.D., Czech Republic)

Virginie Gonzalez-Garcin[1], Gaëlle Soulard[1], Petr Velemínský[2],
Petra Stránská[3] and Jaroslav Bruzek[1,4]

[1]*UMR 5199 PACEA, Anthropologie des Populations Passées et Présentes,*
Université Bordeaux1, Talence,
[2]*Department of Anthropology, National Museum, Prague,*
[3]*Institute of Archaeology, Academy of Sciences of the Czech Republic, Prague,*
[4]*Department of Anthropology, Faculty of Humanities, West Bohemian University, Pilsen,*
[1]*France*
[2,3,4]*Czech Republic*

1. Introduction

Dental growth is recognized to be less influenced by environmental factors than by genetics (Halcrow & Tayles, 2008; Saunders et al., 2000; Scheuer & Black, 2000a). However, it has been demonstrated that dental health is partly conditioned by the differential enamel susceptibility of environmental attack (sugars, bacterial flora, etc.) (Hillson, 1979; Johansson et al., 1994; König & Navia, 1995; Navia, 1994). In an earlier article published in HOMO, 2010, vol. 61, p. 421-439, our results showed that there is some influence of lifestyle on dental health of juvenile individuals (Garcin et al., 2010). Four populations belonged from rural and urban, coastal and inland lifestyles were compared in that paper. We would like, in this chapter, to refine these results with the evaluation of the influence of socioeconomic status on dental health in juvenile individuals with limited dental care. The point of view is focused on tooth development and enamel quality rather than strict caries analyses.

The influence of socioeconomic status on health is a very common topic on living populations (e.g. Alvarez & Navia, 1989; Greksa et al., 2007; Klein and Palmer, 1941; O'Sullivan et al., 1992; Van de Poel et al., 2007). One of the main biases to study these populations is the difficulty to define the environmental framework of the analysis. It is nearly the same in past populations but they have the advantage of the sample size (especially on children). However, most studies on past and historic populations evaluating both dental enamel hypoplasia and caries, are based on adult remains only (Barthelemy et al., 1999; Belcastro et al., 2007; Cucina et al., 2006; Esclassan et al., 2009; Palubeckaité et al.,

2002; Wright, 1997), while it is well accepted that juveniles, and thus their skeletons, are the most sensitive to social and environmental conditions (Bennike et al., 2005; Humphrey & King, 2000; Lewis, 2007; Lewis & Gowland, 2007; Pinhasi et al., 2005). That is why this new study is focused only on juveniles. Several biases must be taken into account with this type of analysis (e.g. Hillson, 2001), but they will be discussed later in the chapter.

We will assess the dental health of juvenile individuals. To be clear till the beginning of this chapter, the main definitions used in this study are given below:

- Enamel hypoplasia is a macroscopically observable quantitative dental defect where enamel thickness has locally decreased on the surfaces of tooth crowns (Clarkson, 1989). As enamel is not remodeled during one's lifetime once it had been formed, hypoplasia provides significant information about stress during development of the dentition (Ubelaker, 1978).
- *"Dental caries may be defined as the localized destruction of tooth tissue by bacterial action"* (Gibbons and van Houte, 1975). Carious lesions lead a process which begins by the enamel surface, and which can conduct, without any care, to the tooth loss (Hillson, 1979). Carious lesions in past populations bring information about their adaptation to their physical and cultural environment (Erdal and Duyar, 1999).
- Both dental traits suffer from the scoring techniques used to evaluate them (Hillson, 2001; Ulijaszek and Lourie, 1997), and comparisons must be careful, when the dental evaluation differs from the samples under study. That is why we have attached a great importance to our methods of recording and analysis.
- Both dental caries and enamel hypoplasia are linked to time (Hillson, 1979; Reich et al., 1999), but in a different way. For dental caries, it is the severity which is the marker of time. Longer the individual will survive; more serious will be the lesion. That is why the age-at-death estimation is important to compare the health state of the juveniles. For dental enamel hypoplasia, the time is important for the moment of appearance of the defect. Thus, it is directly linked to the enamel development. Age-at-death estimation will be used in this way to define when the individuals have suffered from biological stress. This information of time will provide other discussion topics and give different analyses of dental development and care.

The aim of this study is to compare two contrasting populations (upper social class *vs.* middle social class in a settlement in expansion), in order to understand how these biological traits are linked to socioeconomic conditions. Bearing in mind the limitations of such studies, such as the osteological paradox effect (Wood et al., 1992) and some methodological biases (Hillson, 2001), special care has been taken in order to ensure the reproducibility of the results and reliable interpretations. We also would like to discuss the difficulty to differentiate the environmental part from the genetic part in dental mineralization and thus in enamel susceptibility to develop caries and hypoplasias.

2. Materials under study

In anthropological studies, skeletal samples are often limited for reliable statistical comparisons (little sample size), and thus we interpret result with many biases. It is all the more so real when we attempt to compare individuals with different lifestyle and/or socioeconomic status.

In this way, the archaeological site of Mikulčice-Valy (cf. Fig. 1) offers many advantages and the Great Moravian Empire is a specific historical period which allows studying the transition between a rural life and a progressive urbanization.

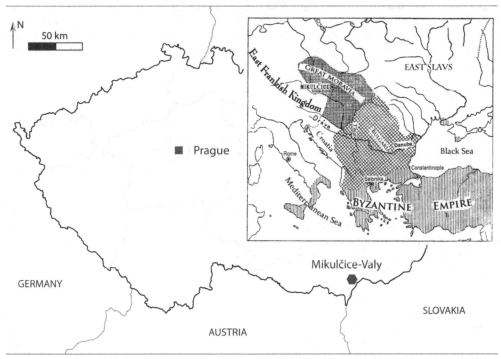

Fig. 1. Situation of the archaeological site under study in relation to current Czech Republic and the location of the Great Moravia in medieval Europe (box adapted from Havelkova et al., 2011).

2.1 Historical background

Till the end of the 8th century, life in Eastern Europe is rather rural with no clear organization and subject to the different waves of migration. Great Moravia was the first Slavic state formation. It was accompanied with a progressive Christianization. The Great Moravian Empire was funded by the Prince Mojmír the 1st (833-846) (Böhm et al., 1963), from different Slavic populations of the northern Danube River. They took advantage from the conflicts between Frankish and Avars in order to found a structured state, bringing together different principalities (Leger, 1868). On the whole, the hierarchic organization is similar to those in Western Europe, with a clear dependency of the peasant farmer to the aristocratic class (Poláček, 2008). With its small territory, the Great Moravian Empire is a privileged area to study the mutation between rural lifestyle to urbanization. Moreover, the principalities are founded around centres of power such as Staré Město, Nitra, or Děvín (Conte, 1986). Mikulčice-Valy was one of these power centres, bringing together the different socioeconomic classes at that time.

2.2 Mikulčice-Valy, how to gather different socioeconomic status in a same archaeological site?

The archaeological site of Mikulčice-Valy is the vastest site in Czech Republic, which is registered as national cultural heritage, and has competed for the World's heritage centre of Unesco since 2001 (http://whc.unesco.org). Situated at 7 km southern from the town Hodonín, near the border of Slovakia, the power centre of Mikulčice was established at the beginning of the 6th century and knew its height between the 9th and 10th centuries (Poláček, 2000; Třeštík, 2001).

2.2.1 The power centre organization

The power centre of Mikulčice is a large fortified settlement, discovered at the end of the 19th century. It is constituted by remains of a palace, at least 12 churches accompanied by several cemeteries, representing more than 2500 burials (Poláček, 2000; Poláček & Marek, 2005; Třeštík, 2001). The remains of the palace were found at the top of some hill above the ancient channel of the Morava River (Fig.2).

The different churches were built around the palace and the basilica (church n°3 on the plan). Archaeological remains suggest that the highest social class (aristocratic part of the population and churchmen) was buried in the cemeteries near these areas. Further the other churches are, lower are the socioeconomic status of the people buried in the adjacent cemeteries.

This organization shows that we could study different social groups in a same site belonging to the same historical period. This is the case and an incredible chance for an anthropological study. However, we must be cautious, because in such settlement moving from urbanization, the limits of each burial place are often difficult to separate and cultural data are missing to exactly differentiate each part of the population. That is why the collections under study come from clear different part of the site in order to have different socioeconomic classes.

2.2.2 Mikulčice "Bazilika", burying the upper social class

The cemetery directly linked to the basilica (named "Bazilika") is of the richest burial place of the area. Many archaeological remains were found suggesting that the upper class was buried here (Poláček et al., 2006). Around the Basilica (IIIrd church) were discovered 564 burials (Poláček, 2008). There are 314 adults, 221 non-adult individuals and 29 individuals with un-estimated age (Stloukal, 1967). The sample under study comprises 217 juvenile individuals (the last four are too poor preserved to be included in the data), ranging from birth to adolescence. In the figures and table, this sample is named Mikulčice Bazilika and is abbreviated "MkB".

2.2.3 Mikulčice "Kostelisko", the suburb of the fortifications

The second area under study is the burial place named "Kostelisko". It takes place in the suburb of the acropolis and is considered as the servants, craftsmen of the castle (Velemínský, 2000; Velemínský et al., 2005). It corresponds to a lower social class than the individuals buried around the basilica. Once again, we must be cautious because of the possible mixture between the parts of the population and the part of the cultural way of thinking that we have no clues.

The second sample under study comprises 425 burials holding 235 juvenile individuals. The skeletons, correctly preserved, present the same age-at-death range than the "Basilika" sample. In the figures and table, this sample is named Mikulčice Kostelisko and is abbreviated "MkK".

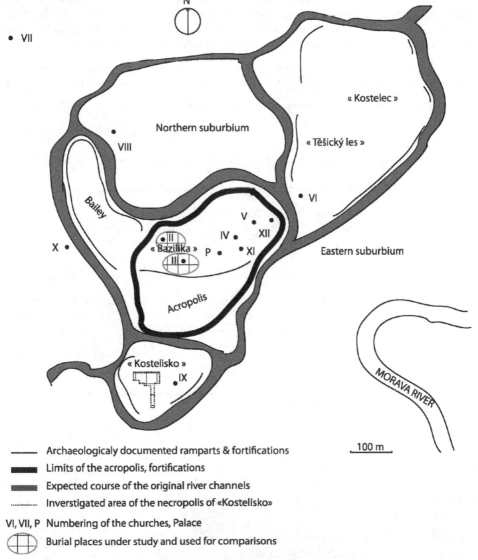

Fig. 2. Mikulčice-Valy, general plan of the site and topography (adapted from Poláček, 2008)

2.2.4 Comparison with other data

The two first samples show contrasting socioeconomic status, whether we consider that the populations were clear separated in the Mikulčice settlement. In order to compare the "urban" samples with a clear different lifestyle, we chose to study a third sample coming from a rural cemetery in the hinterland of Mikulčice.

The archaeological site of Prušánky, is situed at less than 10 km from Mikulčice. This geographical closeness does not reflect proximity in the lifestyle. Indeed, the cemetery associated at this site represents a rural population (Beeby et al., 1982). The location near the power center induces clear exchanges between the two community, but the lifestyle is different. This second site seemed to be self-sufficient (Klanica, 2006a). 676 burials accompanied by Moravian archaeological remains were excavated (Klanica, 2006b).

The last sample under study comprises 173 juvenile individuals from newborn to late adolescent. In the figures and table, this sample is named Prušánky and is abbreviated "Pk".

Thus the three samples show different socioeconomic status:

- MkB, the "aristocratic" and churchmen sample, representing the highest social class of the site;
- MkK, the "middle social class" (above all "craftsmen), who are poorer than the individuals of MkB;
- And Pk, the rural place, where the lifestyle contrasts with the two others.

Their teeth should reflect these life conditions and socioeconomic status. All the skeletal remains are deposited in the Department of Anthropology of the National Museum in Prague.

3. Methods

This study is only based on dental health and lifestyle and on the potential influence of the socioeconomic status on caries prevalence and enamel composition. However, it has been completed by an analysis on the same influence but on bone growth and composition.

The resulting dental sample consists of 6123 observed teeth. Table 1 gives the details for each sample.

3.1 Recording dental health and defects

In dental stress and caries assessment it is clearly desirable to record the least subjective stages and observations, in order to minimize the intra- and inter-observer errors (Danforth et al., 1993), both of which are often significant. The intra- and inter-observer error, for the protocol proposed below, has been tested and has been published in a previous paper (Garcin et al. 2010). As the protocol is the same in this study, we do not remind the results but we expose the features quoted and the statistical procedures employed for comparisons.

Both dental caries and enamel hypoplasia have been recorded because they give different information on enamel susceptibility to develop lesions. International dental charts were used to identify the teeth (such as n° 18 to 11 for upper right permanent teeth).

Sample	Deciduous teeth	Permanent teeth	Total
MkB	894	651	1545
MkK	1103	1790	2893
Pk	823	862	1685
Total	2820	3303	**6123**

Table 1. Tooth samples for each site

3.1.1 Dental caries

The presence of caries was scored in all tooth types that is to say on deciduous and permanent teeth when detected macroscopically. When there was a doubt on caries development because of the tooth preservation, the development of the lesion was tested by a dental probe.

Four features were observed and scored for the lesions:

- The number of caries per tooth;
- The area & side where the lesion occurred: occlusal, buccal, lingual or interproximal lesions.
- The location of the lesion on the anatomical tooth: the root, the cement-enamel junction (also referred as cervical region or neck), and the crown;
- And finally, the severity of the lesion was quoted on a three-stages scale (fig. 3):
  - Stage 1: small lesion which affects only the enamel and less than 10% of the tooth surface;
  - Stage 2: medium lesion which affects both enamel and dentin and spread from 10% to 50% of the tooth surface;
  - Stage 3: large lesions penetrating all the dental tissues, enamel, dentin and pulp. They take more than 50% of the tooth surface.

These simple stages are easy to define, thus the results of scoring would be less prone to errors, because in archaeological record there are some cases of complex observations (Hillson, 2001), even if we cannot totally avoid subjectivity in such study. This subjectivity is all the more right when we attempt to analyze dental enamel hypoplasia.

3.1.2 Dental enamel hypoplasia

Hypoplastic defects occur in three forms: linear, pitting and plane. However, their expression is different on deciduous and permanent dentition (Lukacs et al., 2001a; Lukacs et al., 2001b; Ogden et al., 2007). We chose to take into consideration the enamel hypoplasia only on the permanent teeth for the quoted features. Nevertheless, a paragraph in the results will be devoted to the different expressions of enamel hypoplasia on deciduous teeth. The presence of macroscopically observed enamel hypoplasia was noted in all types of permanent teeth.

Four characteristics have been recorded:

- The number of hypoplasia per tooth;
- The type of hypoplasia: linear, pitting or plane;
- The severity of the defect on a three-stages scale (only for linear defects) (fig. 4):

- Stage 1: the defect is macroscopically detectable, but is less than 0.1mm width;
- Stage 2: the defect is obvious, but the enamel is not distorted around the line;
- Stage 3: is the most severe with formation of shoving on the enamel surface;
- The location of the defect is the third of the affected crown: cemento-enamel junction third, middle third or occlusal third.

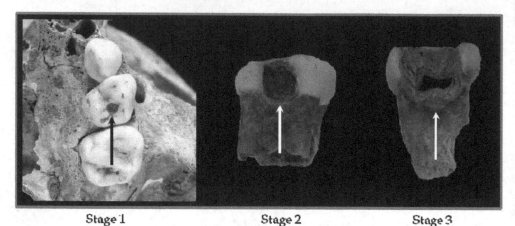

Stage 1   Stage 2   Stage 3

Fig. 3. Illustration of the three-stage severity scale for scoring dental caries (photos: V. Gonzalez-Garcin)

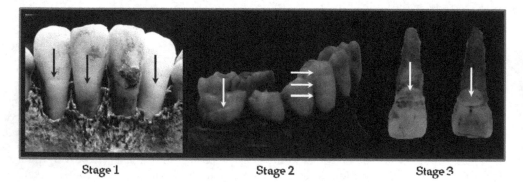

Stage 1   Stage 2   Stage 3

Fig. 4. Illustration of the three-stage severity scale for scoring dental enamel hypoplasia (photos: V. Gonzalez-Garcin)

The distance between the cement-enamel junction and the defect for the calculation of the time of appearance of the defect (Reid & Dean, 2000), was not taken because we only made macroscopical analysis. Charts relative to age differ according to different authors and thus mineralization is not really taken into account. In such large studies, with this method the stages cannot provide accurate chronological sequences (Fitzgerald & Saunders, 2005; Hillson & Bond, 1997; Ritzman et al., 2008). However, a global chart has been made in order to evaluate which developmental stage is the most concerned by enamel hypoplasia.

3.2 Estimating age-at-death

In archaeological samples, the first step for anthropological studies is the age-at-death estimation. This estimation will be useful to compare the different sites, because, dentition is also related to age. Currently, the most reliable methods to estimate an age are those based on dental mineralization and developmental stages (Boldsen et al., 2002; Ritz-Timme et al., 2000; Scheuer & Black, 2000b; Schmitt, 2005). We chose to estimate age-at-death in our sample with the method of Moorrees et al. (1963a,b), because we are working on teeth and we wanted a uniform method and no combination of several methods. Moreover, we just needed some different stages to compare our sites, that is why we classified the individuals in 5 age classes (usually used in historical demography): 0, 5-9, 10-14, and 15-19 years.

A last comparison has been made using the dental mineralization sequences. This approach use the mineralization stages of Moorrees et al. (1963a,b), as a base for determining a dental sequence. These basic sequences (one for each individual) are in a second time grouped following the big tooth developmental phases in order to simplify the data (many combinations are possible). Six final groups are defined and used for comparison:

- Group 1: from the beginning of deciduous crown formation to the end of the emergence of all deciduous teeth;
- Group 2: latency period of deciduous teeth. The permanent incisors and the first permanent molars complete their crown formation.
- Group 3: this group corresponds to the mixed dentition. The first deciduous teeth are replaced by permanent incisors (most standard sequence). The first molar emerges anatomically*. This is the first step of permanent teeth emergence.
- Group 4: stability period where the roots of permanent teeth (incisors and first molars) complete their formation. The roots of the other teeth just initialize their mineralization.
- Group 5: secondary phase of tooth emergence for permanent canine, premolars and second molars.
- Group 6: completion of the permanent dentition (except third molars which were not taken into account.

The illustration of the six resulting groups is presented in fig. 5.

3.3 Statistical procedures

The analyses were performed in three steps. First, in order in order to calculate the frequencies of dental enamel hypoplasia, the total number of available teeth, fully erupted and/or isolated, has been used for observation. Tooth germs in both the mandible and maxilla were not taken into account. With the same objective, frequencies of dental caries were calculated using only the teeth in occlusion. The usual calibrations (Erdal & Duyar, 1999; Hillson, 2001; Lukacs, 1995) adjusting the proportions of tooth type and *ante mortem* tooth loss were applied.

In a second time, inter-population comparisons were conducted using the non-parametric χ^2 statistical. Finally, we studied the interrelationship between caries and hypoplastic defects

---

* The emergence is a localized phenomenon, which corresponds to the appearance of the tooth in the mouth. We distinguish the clinical emergence where the tooth pierces the gingival tissue from the anatomical emergence where the tooth passes over the alveolar bone.

in order to evaluate the role of enamel structure on caries development. All statistical procedures and calculations were carried out by using Statsoft® Statistica version 7.1 and Microsoft® Office Excel 2007.

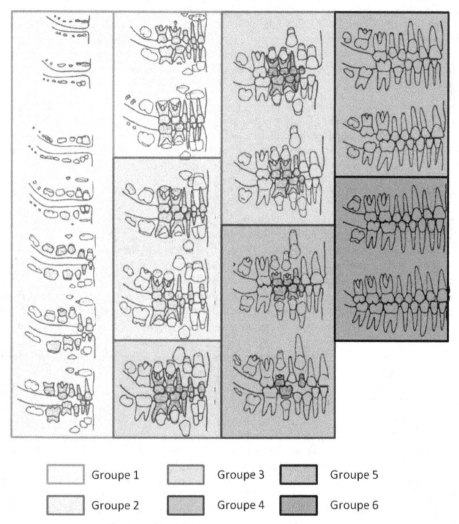

Groupe 1   Groupe 3   Groupe 5

Groupe 2   Groupe 4   Groupe 6

Fig. 5. Representation of the established groups from the dental mineralization sequences (adapted from Ubelaker, 1978)

4. Results

As mentioned in our previous paper, intra- and inter-observers errors must be taken into account, but although they have an impact on the results, those are always discussed with these biases (Garcin et al. 2010).

4.1 Prevalence of dental caries

Frequencies of caries in all observable teeth are presented in figure 6 & 7. The evaluated teeth are those observable in the oral cavity and/or in occlusion. This information is different for dental enamel hypoplasia, because tooth germs, when isolated, were also evaluated for this second dental trait.

As often mentioned, posterior teeth are more affected than anterior teeth, which confirm the differential susceptibility of the molars to be suffering from dental caries (Klein & Palmer, 1941; Oyamada et al., 2008; Saunders et al., 1997). But it is interesting to point out that some individuals are attained by carious lesions on anterior deciduous teeth in both area of Mikulčice. These lesions are often related to higher enamel susceptibility to develop dental caries, even on permanent teeth (Li & Wang, 2002; O'Sullivan & Tinanoff, 1993).

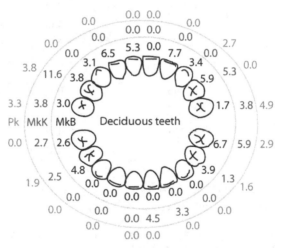

Fig. 6. Caries frequencies per tooth type in the three collections (deciduous dentition)

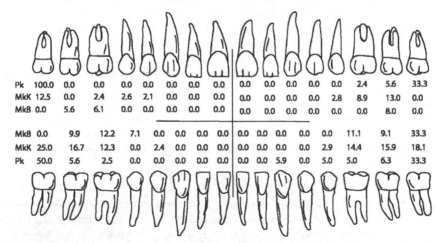

Pk	100.0	0.0	0.0	0.0	0.0	0.0	0.0	0.0	0.0	0.0	0.0	0.0	0.0	2.4	5.6	33.3
MkK	12.5	0.0	2.4	2.6	2.1	0.0	0.0	0.0	0.0	0.0	0.0	0.0	2.8	8.9	13.0	0.0
MkB	0.0	5.6	6.1	0.0	0.0	0.0	0.0	0.0	0.0	0.0	0.0	0.0	0.0	0.0	8.0	0.0

MkB	0.0	9.9	12.2	7.1	0.0	0.0	0.0	0.0	0.0	0.0	0.0	0.0	0.0	11.1	9.1	33.3
MkK	25.0	16.7	12.3	0.0	2.4	0.0	0.0	0.0	0.0	0.0	0.0	0.0	2.9	14.4	15.9	18.1
Pk	50.0	5.6	2.5	0.0	0.0	0.0	0.0	0.0	0.0	0.0	5.9	0.0	5.0	5.0	6.3	33.3

Fig. 7. Caries frequencies per tooth type in the three collections (permanent dentition)

In terms of global calibrated prevalence, there is a difference between the Mikulčice areas and Prušánky in the caries frequencies on both deciduous and permanent teeth. The frequency of dental caries in the deciduous and permanent teeth from Prušánky was statistically significantly lower (χ^2 = 4.49; p = 0.03 for permanent teeth and χ^2 = 9.08; p < 0.01 for deciduous teeth) than in those from the two other collections. Table 2 shows the prevalence and the comparisons between features in the three collections.

	Mikulčice Bazilika	Mikulčice Kostelisko	Prušánky
Prevalence on deciduous teeth	0.03	0.03	**0.01**
Prevalence on permanent teeth	0.03	0.04	**0.02**
Location of the lesions			
Occlusal – crown	0.36	0.34	0.52
Interproximal – crown	0.24	0.15	**0.11**
Interproximal – crown & neck	0.25	0.19	**0.11**
Large caries (more than 2/3 of the tooth affected)	**0.02**	0.09	0.15
Other locations	0.13	0.23	0.11
Severity of the lesions			
1	0.51	0.57	0.40
2	0.45	0.34	0.44
3	0.04	0.09	**0.13**

Table 2. Caries prevalence and differences in caries descriptive features between the three collections (statistically significant differences are in bold)

Concerning the lesions traits, the most common are the occlusal caries in all sites. Once again, the site of Prušánky differs from the others. Indeed, there are less interproximal lesions in this collection than in the others (χ^2 = 8.48; p < 0.03 for the crown and χ^2 = 8.70; p < 0.03). Furthermore, another significant difference is shown for the severity of the lesion. But this time, the trend is reversed. Individuals of Mikulčice Bazilika have less severe lesions (stage 3) than in the two other collections (χ^2 = 8.63; p < 0.03). The large caries are less frequent in Mikulčice Bazilika individuals. Prušánky's individual are the most affected. Is there a relationship between the severity of the lesions, the diet, and/or the dental care? This notion will be discussed later. Apart this last trait, we can observe that individuals from the two areas of Mikulčice have very similar features even if their socioeconomic status differs. The rural lifestyle seems to have more impact on dental health than socioeconomic status. The tooth development is also very important in the comprehension of the caries susceptibility. That is why dental enamel hypoplasia will give another type of information.

4.2 Expression of the dental enamel hypoplasia

Contrary to the caries, dental enamel hypoplasia have been observed on all permanent teeth, even tooth germs. They will give information on crown development. Before discussing the differences between the collections, a paragraph on hypoplasia on deciduous teeth summarizes the encountered cases.

4.2.1 Dental enamel hypoplasia on deciduous canines

Dental enamel hypoplasia on deciduous teeth were observed on four individuals from
Mikulčice Bazilika. Any other individual presents hypoplasia in the other collections. All the
cases correspond to what is named "localised enamel hypoplasia of human deciduous
canines" (Clarkson, 1989; Taji et al., 2000). The figure 8 shows some of the observed cases.

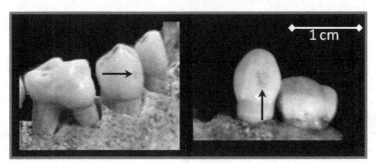

Fig. 8. Illustration of two localized enamel hypoplasia on deciduous lower canines

Some discussions exist on the aetiology of this sort of enamel defect (Skinner & Hung, 1989;
Sweeney et al., 1971): genotype or environment? This point will be taken back in the next part
of the chapter. All defects are localized on lower canine and are bilateral on 50% of the cases.
The two unilateral cases show less marked than the bilateral ones. These four cases give
argument for the difference of enamel susceptibility following the socioeconomic status.

4.2.2 Results on dental enamel hypoplasia on permanent teeth

We took into account only linear enamel hypoplasia (LEH), because pitting defects were
defeated (less than 2% in each collection, 0% at Mikulčice Bazilika). The comparison of LEH
global prevalences between collections show a significant difference between Mikulčice's
areas, and Prušánky (Table 3).

	Mikulčice Bazilika	Mikulčice Kostelisko	Prušánky
Total prevalence	**0.12**	0.18	0.16
Frequency of individuals affected (%)	10.59	**30.63**	17.91
Severity			
1	0.63	0.52	**0.29**
2	0.32	0.47	**0.61**
3	0.05	0.01	0.10
Part of the affected crown (beginning from the cervical region)			
Proximal third	0.21	0.29	0.34
Mesial third	0.59	0.55	0.57
Distal third	0.15	0.14	0.09
Whole height of the crown	0.04	0.02	0.00

Table 3. Linear enamel hypoplasia prevalence and differences in defect descriptive features
between the three collections (statistically significant differences are in bold)

The whole prevalence (taking into account all observed teeth) is significantly lower in Mikulčice Bazilika (χ^2 = 8.61; p < 0.03). If we consider the frequency of individuals affected, the greatest frequency is at Mikulčice Kostelisko with more than 30% of individuals (χ^2 = 9.81; p < 0.01). If we consider the prevalence per tooth type, the results are given by the figure 9.

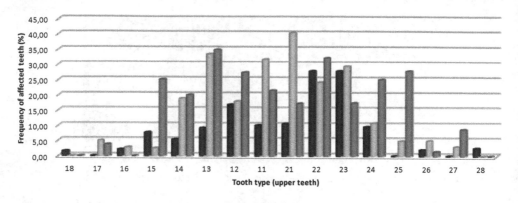

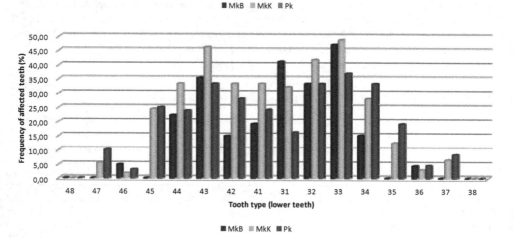

Fig. 9. Frequency of enamel hypoplasia per tooth type in the three collections

These graphs clearly show that there is a differential susceptibility in tooth type for developing LEH (Goodman & Armelagos, 1985; Palubeckaité et al., 2002; Wright, 1997). Anterior teeth (incisors & canines) are more affected by the defect than posterior teeth (premolars & molars). On the whole, canines are the most affected. Even if differences between sites could be shown, they are not statistically significant (number of teeth per tooth type differs, thus graphic results are misleading). We can see that posterior teeth are also affected, demonstrated that these individuals suffered from non specific stress during late infancy period, that is to say during the time of formation of posterior tooth crowns. This point is important for the next paragraph concerning the relationship between the lesions, the defects, and the age-at-death.

Concerning the other features, the severity of the defects are obviously the same in the two areas of Mikulčice. The trend is inverted for Prušánky. There are more medium defects (stage 2) than slight defects (stage 1) in this collection ($\chi^2 = 14.16$; $p < 0.01$ & $\chi^2 = 20.15$; $p < 0.01$). Once again, the lifestyle seems to be more expressed by dental stress than the socioeconomic status. But what is more surprising is that this is the only feature which differs from the others. On the whole, the three collections present the same trend in LEH expression.

The last information given by table 3, is that the part of the affected crown does not show any statistical difference ($p > 0.05$ for all statistical tests). This means that there is globally no difference on the period when the biological stress arose. The specific study with age estimation gives other information. Few individuals present teeth with all the crown height affected by multiple LEH. The stress period are thus isolated and occurred seldom more than two times during the crown formation. The next part presents when this stress took place in the crown formation, and its relationship with age-at-death.

4.2.3 Age influence and relationship between caries lesions and hypoplastic defects

Two approaches were lead to evaluate the age influence on dental health and development:

- The first one is the representation of the mean age when the stress occurred (on lower permanent teeth). Figure 10 show these periods of stress for each collection. The data were calculated from those of Reid and Dean (2000) and Skinner & Goodman (1992). We also used the records on the affected third (table 3). Only the highest frequency is mentioned in order to leave the figure readable. This figure takes into account only the crown mineralization, thus the stress which is arisen during puberty is not mentioned.

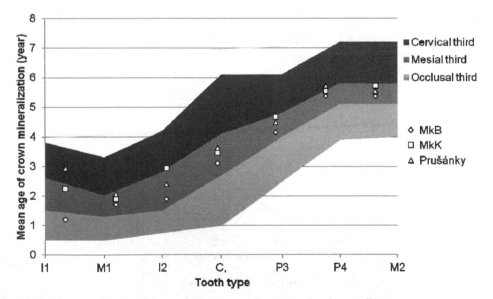

Fig. 10. Frequency of enamel hypoplasia per tooth type in the three collections

- It is noticeable that few stress arose during the occlusal third mineralization (light grey), apart for the first incisor in Mikulčice Bazilika. The individuals were subjected to stress during infancy, and especially between 2 and 6 years, and the stress concerns mainly the mesial third of the crowns for all collections. These results can be transposed to upper teeth. There is no statistical difference between collections for these stress periods (p>0.05 for all statistical tests). Even if this approach is not very precise, it gives a good mean of comparison. Here, Mikulčice Bazilika seems to be different because the stress periods arose sooner in the mineralization stages than in the other collections. If we compare now the prevalence of dental lesions and defects in age classes, the frequencies are represented in figure 11.

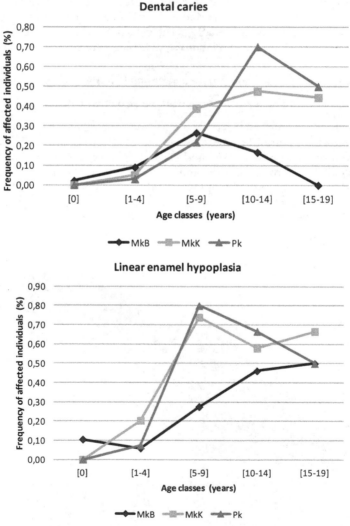

Fig. 11. Frequency of dental caries, and linear enamel hypoplasia per age class

When we compare the three collections by age class, it is noteworthy to remark that the individuals of Mikulčice Bazilika differ from the others for the classes 10-14, and 15-19 years for the caries lesions and for the class 5-9 for the LEH. Frequencies are significantly different between sites ($p < 0.05$). For the dental caries, it should be an evidence of a better dental care in higher socioeconomic status populations. For LEH, less individuals are affected during the juvenile period, is the environment less stressing in higher socioeconomic status? These points will be discussed in the next part.

The second approach compares the dental features according to the tooth mineralization sequences describe in the methods. It is another mean to precise the last results, without using age estimation but biological traits. Table 4 gives the comparison for both dental caries & LEH.

These more biological data (we avoid age-at-death estimation) confirm precedent results, giving significant differences for the individuals of Mikulčice Bazilika in both dental caries and LEH. Indeed, the group 5 and 6 of Mikulčice Bazilika are significantly less affected by caries lesions than those of Mikulčice Kostelisko and Prušánky. The last graph gave a trend; here we have a reliable result. We also notice a difference in group 4 and 5 for the LEH. The arguments of dental care and attenuated stress for these stages of development are thus strengthened.

Group	Mikulčice Bazilika		Mikulčice Kostelisko		Prušánky	
	Caries	LEH	Caries	LEH	Caries	LEH
1	0.00%	5.26%	0.00%	8.82%	0.00%	0.00%
2	7.14%	23.08%	4.17%	22.73%	10.52%	21.05%
3	27.27%	41.67%	31.82%	57.14%	27.27%	36.36%
4	20.00%	**20.00%**	25.00%	90.90%	20.00%	80.00%
5	**11.11%**	**55.56%**	50.00%	78.13%	23.07%	78.57%
6	**0.00%**	62.46%	88.89%	73.68%	61.53%	61.53%

Table 4. Frequency of dental caries, and linear enamel hypoplasia per dental mineralization group (significant differences are in bold)

To sum up, few differences between the collections are highlighted: one on global prevalence of LEH, and two on location and severity of dental caries. However, if we compare more biological traits, related to tooth development and enamel susceptibility, then, some trends to discuss appear.

5. Discussion

Three main topics will be discussed in this last part. The first one deals with the assets and the drawbacks of archaeological collections in a study of dental health. The second develops the influence of socioeconomic status on dental mineralization. And finally, we will discuss the differential enamel susceptibility to be affected from defects and lesions.

5.1 Archaeological collections: assets and drawbacks in the study of socioeconomic influence on dental health

There are many studies on the influence of lifestyle and/or socioeconomic status on dental health (Bodoriková et al., 2005; Duray, 1990; Kim & Durden, 2007; Vodanovic et al., 2005). However, they concern both living and past populations. Moreover, the protocol of observation and statistical analyses differ from one to another. Thus, it is very difficult to compare the results and to be confident in our interpretations. That is why we chose to work only on huge archaeological samples, even if they also have some downsides. The tooth sample size in archaeological collections are mostly important (several hundreds of teeth), especially for medieval cemeteries. Large burials places are excavated, giving many individuals, including juveniles. The sample size is sufficient to provide reliable statistical results. Nevertheless, regarding the bone and teeth preservation, data are as often as not missing, and we do not have all dentition for each individual (Duyar & Erdal, 2003; Hillson, 2001). That is why different calibrations are calculated to adjust the frequencies and to take into account the missing data.

The second advantage of archaeological collection is that we can have homogeneous collections, that is to say that population of a same cemetery comes from a global same lifestyle and the admixture (thus the influence of genetic part) is less pronounced than in living population. However, in such collection, we have the problem of age-at-death estimation. When studies based on living populations have accurate age of the subjects under study, in our case estimations (even with reliable methods) give at best age classes (Albert and Greene, 1999; Cole, 2003; Heuzé & Cardoso, 2008; Lewis & Gowland, 2007). This study uses a little the age-at-death estimation that is why we try to free from this bias using dental mineralization stages. The obtained results and differences highlighted show that this is a way to work to enhance the quality and reliability of our study.

The third point to discuss also deals with reliability, but on the recording methods. It has been mentioned in the second part of this chapter that we have evaluated the intra- and inter-observer error of our protocol for both caries lesions and enamel hypoplasia. To go back on the terms of Ulijaszek & Lourie (1997), we must compare something comparable. Yet, recording dental caries and enamel hypoplasia is always a little bit subjective. The data must be as quantitative as possible and thus at least qualitative (Landis & Koch, 1977). The results of intra- and inter-observer errors in our last study (Garcin et al., 2010), show that even if the results are satisfactory, we cannot completely be completely free from this bias (Berti & Mahaney, 1995; Danforth et al., 1993; Hillson, 1992).

Being aware from these main biases, we can discuss the influence of socioeconomic status on dental health and development.

5.2 Have you spoken of a possible socioeconomic influence on dental health and development?

Our results show that except an inferior global prevalence of LEH and less invading caries in the higher socioeconomic status collection, there is no difference between the individuals of Mikulčice. On the other hand, Prušánky individuals differ from the other more often, especially on dental caries. Do these results intend that the lifestyle have more influence on dental health than the socioeconomic status? We explained in the materials paragraph that it is quite difficult to define a clear socioeconomic status in archaeological populations even if they are relative homogeneous. To answer clearly this question in the big site of Mikulčice, it should be interesting to compare all parts of the area. However, comparing the prevalence of LEH in other mediaeval/modern groups in Europe (Coulon et al., 2008; Herold, 2008; Šlaus et al., 2002) it is apparent that our values are relatively low, but overall features are similar to the other studies. It is the same for the caries lesions even if the results are hardly comparable (Espeland et al., 1988; Rudney et al., 1983; Watt et al., 1997; Williams & Curzon, 1985). Nevertheless, our results counteract several other studies (on past and present populations), which claim that the socioeconomic status influence the health (Goodman et al., 1988; Hauser, 1994; Henneberg et al., 2001; Kim & Durden, 2007). Although a direct parallel is difficult, this is a striking result. We must keep in mind the limits of such studies and thus accept that we give only trends, especially on the relationship between the dental development and the socioeconomic status. To our point of view, in past population, we should take into account the global lifestyle rather than searching to define a clear socioeconomic status. Besides we found in our last studies clear differences between rural and urban lifestyle, what was confirmed by many studies (Betsinger, 2007; Budnik & Liczbinska, 2006; Riva et al., 2009; Van de Poel et al., 2007; Williams & Galley, 1995). We also must take in mind that in past population, we must deal with the "osteological paradox" (Byers, 1994; Wood et al., 1992; Wright & Yoder, 2003). The juvenile individuals we study are those who have not survived and who have never reached the adulthood (Saunders & Hoppa, 1993). On the contrary, the individuals showing dental defects and lesions survived sufficiently a long time to develop the trait we wanted to record. Thus, healthy past populations are not necessarily those who the most suffer from biological stress and who had the best dental care. That is why it is interesting to focus on biological traits only, avoiding abusive interpretations. The relationship between dental development and health seem to be a good track to go into in depth.

5.3 Dental mineralization, enamel susceptibility, and health

Until now, relatively few studies have considered the possible relationship between enamel hypoplasia and dental caries (Khan et al., 1999; Schneider, 1986; Sweeney et al., 1969; Walker & Hewlett, 1990). Even if tooth susceptibility is different for the two indicators, we could imagine that enamel with defects is more sensible to bacterial attacks. This hypothesis was examined by establishing a chart given the frequency by age class having one of the traits or both traits under study (Table 5).

This table clearly shows that there is slight correlation between caries and hypoplasia. Indeed, the individuals of Mikulčice Kostelisko and Prušánky can develop both traits in the same time but it is not a sweeping statement. Only older age classes (after 5 years old) show the possible relationship, but most of the defects and lesions appear separately. What is striking is that the individuals having the localized hypoplasia on deciduous teeth also have LEH on permanent teeth, and also caries lesions. This caries susceptibility seem to be related to hypocalcified teeth (Duray, 1990), and repeated stress periods. This observation was also made in several studies, but not only on human but also in Great Apes (Lukacs, 1999a; Lukacs, 1999b; Lukacs, 2001; Skinner & Goodman, 1992). Moreover, most of the authors link this observation to a low nutritional status (Norén, 1983; Skinner & Hung, 1989; Sweeney et al., 1971; Taji et al., 2000). Even if genetics mainly lead dental development, the environmental conditions and stress periods also influence the dental mineralization and thus the enamel susceptibility to be affected by caries. Even if it is difficult to demonstrate, it seems that after passing a certain threshold, the underlying aetiological factors resulting in caries and enamel hypoplasia interact, creating a vicious cycle – physiological balance is disturbed through pathogens and inadequate nutrition, compromising metabolism and the immune system. This makes the afflicted individual susceptible to further infections and ultimately even more unable to cope with additional stresses (Obertova, 2005; Obertova &

Thurzo, 2008). This last remark corroborates our comparisons with the biological groups, which show that juveniles are more likely to develop both traits on permanent teeth.

Even if this study raises only some trends and being aware of its limits, we do not want misinterpret, the relation to age and indirect influence of the socioeconomic status on defects and lesions are obvious. We must find now the methodological and theoretical framework to prove them.

6. Conclusion

The goal of the present research was to obtain information about the influence of the socioeconomic status on dental health and development by determining the prevalence and characteristics of enamel hypoplasia and caries in two Great Moravian populations at Mikulčice and Prušánky.

Collection / Age group	CAR0 / LEH0		CAR1 / LEH1		CAR1 / LEH0		CAR0 / LEH1		Total
	n	Frequency	n	Frequency	n	Frequency	n	Frequency	
Mikulčice Bazilika									
0	41	**0.85**	0	0.00	1	0.02	6	0.13	48
1-4	83	**0.83**	0	0.00	9	0.09	8	0.08	100
5-9	24	**0.70**	1	0.03	8	0.24	1	0.03	34
10-14	12	**0.66**	1	0.06	2	0.11	3	0.17	18
15-19	6	**1.00**	0	0.00	0	0.00	0	0.00	6
ND	10	**0.91**	0	0.00	0	0.00	1	0.09	11
Total	176	**0.81**	2	0.01	20	0.09	19	0.09	217
Mikulčice Kostelisko									
0	36	**1.00**	0	0.00	0	0.00	0	0.00	36
1-4	63	**0.82**	3	0.04	1	0.01	10	0.13	77
5-9	15	0.28	20	**0.37**	1	0.02	18	0.33	54
10-14	8	**0.38**	8	**0.38**	2	0.10	3	0.14	21
15-19	2	0.22	3	**0.33**	1	0.11	3	**0.33**	9
ND	31	0.25	1	0.25	1	0.25	1	0.25	4
Total	155	**0.66**	35	0.15	6	0.03	35	0.15	231
Prušánky									
0	48	**1.00**	0	0.00	0	0.00	0	0.00	48
1-4	59	**0.91**	0	0.00	2	0.03	4	0.06	65
5-9	11	0.36	6	0.19	1	0.03	14	**0.44**	32
10-14	2	0.20	5	**0.50**	2	0.20	1	0.10	10
15-19	0	0.00	0	0.00	1	**0.50**	1	**0.50**	2
ND	16	**1.00**	0	0.00	0	0.00	0	0.00	16
Total	136	**0.79**	11	0.06	6	0.03	36	0.12	173

CAR 0: absence of caries; CAR 1: presence of caries; LEH 0: absence of hypoplasia; LEH 1: presence of linear hypoplasia; ND: non defined age-at-death.

Table 5. Prevalence of caries against LEH per age group in the three collections (the highest frequencies are in bold)

Dental analysis revealed a slightly influence of socioeconomic status on dental health. In addition, considering the observed prevalence of the hypoplastic lesions and caries in the analysed skeletal samples, a pattern emerged suggestive of probable influence of lifestyle and high importance of studying biological traits rather than using age-at-death estimation.

Two main prospects are highlighted from this research: the need of analyzing the whole sample of Mikulčice-Valy in order to compare other socioeconomic status in big dental samples, and integrated new methods in population studies to avoid abusive interpretations and more reliable comparisons. The large sample size of juveniles and preservation of the skeletal material make the early medieval Great Moravian populations at Mikulčice and Prušanky unique in their ability to demonstrate the distribution of two dental indicators, dental caries and enamel hypoplasia. We are convinced that the study of non-adult skeletal and dental remains is one of the best mean to increase our knowledge of the environmental and genetic parts in the human development, and certainly one of the most challenging and exciting area of research in Physical Anthropology and Bioarchaeology.

7. Acknowledgment

We thank M. Bessou, and M. Jantač for their assistance with various phases of this study, especially for the radiographs used in dental age estimation. We also thank the Horní Počernice warehouse team and the National Museum of Prague for its welcome at each mission. Statistical analysis for the software of age-at-death estimation was carried out by V. Honkimaki (ESRF, Grenoble), and without him, the new approach would never have been developed. Thanks also go to P. Sellier, and L. Poláček for their discussions on historical background, and on dental defect scoring. We are also grateful to Mrs. Batby for reading and commenting on the manuscript. Special thanks to my husband for his help with the images processing. To all of these people and institutions we are immensely grateful.

8. References

Albert, A. & Greene, D. (1999). Bilateral Asymetry in Skeletal Growth and Maturation as an Indicator of Environmental Stress. *American Journal of Physical Anthropology*, Vol.110, No.3, (November 1999), pp. 341-349, ISSN 1096-8644

Alvarez, J. & Navia, J. (1989). Nutritional status, tooth eruption, and dental caries: A review. *American Journal of Clinical Nutrition*, Vol.49, No.3, (March 1989), pp. 417-426, ISSN 0002-9165

Barthelemy, I.; Telmont, N.; Crubézy, E. & Rouge, D. (1999). Etude de la pathologie stomatologique et maxillo-faciale dans une population médiévale (Xe - XII e siècles) du sud-ouest de la France. *Revue de Stomatologie et de Chirurgie Maxillo-Faciale*, Vol.100, No.3, (June 1999), pp. 133-139, ISSN 0035-1768

Beeby, S.; Buckton, D. & Klanica Z. (1982). *Great Moravia: The Archaeology of Ninth-Century Czechoslovakia*, British Museum Publications, ISBN 978-071-4105-20-8, Londres, United Kingdom

Belcastro, G.; Rastelli, E.; Mariotti, V.; Consiglio, C.; Facchini, F. & Bonfiglioli, B. (2007). Continuity or Discontinuity of the Life-Style in the Central Italy During the Roman Imperial Age-Early Middle Ages Transition: Diet, Health, and Behavior. *American*

Journal of Physical Anthropology, Vol.132, No.3, (March 2007), pp. 381-394, ISSN 1096-8644

Bennike, P.; Lewis, M.E.; Schutkowski, H. & Valentin, F. (2005). Comparison of Child Morbidity in Two Contrasting Medieval Cemeteries From Denmark. *American Journal of Physical Anthropology*, Vol. 128, No.4, (December 2005), pp. 734-746, ISSN 1096-8644

Berti, P. & Mahaney, M. (1995). Conservative Scoring and Exclusion of the Phenomenon of Interest in Linear Enamel Hypoplasia Studies. *American Journal of Human Biology*, Vol.7, No.3, (May 1995), pp. 313-320, ISSN 1520-6300

Betsinger, T. (2007). *The Biological Consequences of Urbanization in Medieval Poland*, The Ohio State University, Ph.D Thesis Dissertation, Colombus, USA

Bodorikova, S.; Thurzo, M. & Drozdova, E. (2005). Kazivost' zubov adolescentov a dospelých zo staroslovanského pohrebiska Pohansko –"Pohřebiště okolo kostela" pri Breclavi, Česka republika. *Acta Rer. Natur. Mus. Nat. Slov.*, Vol.51, pp. 88–101

Böhm, J.; Havránek, B.; Kolejka, J.; & Poulík, J. (1963). *La Grande-Moravie: tradition millénaire de l'État et de la civilisation*, Éditions de l'Académie Tchécoslovaque des Sciences, ISBN 702-691-0968-81-3, Prague, Czech Republic

Boldsen, J.; Milner, G.; Konigsberg, L. & Wood, J. (2002). Transition analysis: a new method for estimating age from skeletons, In: *Paleodemography. Age distributions from skeletal samples*, R.D. Hoppa & J.W. Vaupel (Eds.), 73-106, Cambridge University Press, ISBN 978-052-1800-63-1, Cambridge, United Kingdom

Budnik, A. & Liczbinska, G. (2006). Urban and Rural Differences in Mortality and Causes of Death in Historical Poland. *American Journal of Physical Anthropology*, Vol.129, No.2, (February 2006), pp. 294-304, ISSN 1096-8644

Byers, S.N. (1994). On stress and stature in the "Osteological Paradox". *Current Anthropology*, Vol.35, No.3, (June 1994), pp. 282-284, ISSN 0011-3204

Clarkson, J. (1989). Review of terminology, classifications, and indices of developmental defects of enamel. *Advances in Dental Research*, Vol.3, No.2, (September 1989), pp. 104-109, ISSN 0022-0345

Cole, T.J. (2003). The secular trend in human physical growth: a biological view. *Economics and Human Biology*, Vol.1, No.2, (June 2003), pp. 161-168, ISSN 1570-677X

Conte, F. (1986). *Les Slaves : aux origines des civilisations d'Europe centrale et orientale : VIe-XIIIe siècles*, Albin Michel, ISBN 978-222-6026-06-4, Paris, France

Coulon, A.; Grimoud, A.M.; Sevin, A. & Paya, D. (2008). Palaeo-epidemiological study of linear enamel hypoplasia in an urban medieval population (4th to 16th century) from the south-west of France: the Toulouse collection of "Saint Michel". *Bulletins et Mémoires de la Société d'Anthropolologie de Paris*, Vol.20, No.3-4, (juillet 2008), pp. 223, ISSN 0037-8984

Cucina, A.; Vargiu, R.; Mancinelli, D.; Ricci, R.; Santandrea, E.; Catalano, P. & Coppa, A. (2006). The Necropolis of Vallerano (Rome, 2nd-3rd Century AD): An Anthropological Perspective on the Ancient Romans in the *Suburbium. International Journal of Osteoarchaeology*, Vol.16, No.2, (March-April 2006), pp.104-117, ISSN 1099-1212

Danforth, M.; Shuler Herndon, K. & Propst, K. (1993). A Preliminary Study of Patterns of Replication in Scoring Linear Enamel Hypoplasias. *International Journal of Osteoarchaeology*, Vol.3, No.2, (June 1993), pp. 297-302, ISSN 1099-1212

Duray, S.M. (1990). Deciduous Enamel Defects and Caries Susceptibility in a Prehistoric Ohio Population. *American Journal of Physical Anthropology*, Vol.81, No.1, (January 1990), pp. 27-34, ISSN 1096-8644

Duyar, I. & Erdal, Y.S. (2003). A new approach for calibrating dental caries frequency of skeletal remains. *Homo*, Vol.54, No.1, (January 2003), pp. 57-70, ISSN 0018-442X

Erdal, Y.S. & Duyar, I. (1999). Brief Communication: A New Correction Procedure for Calibrating Dental Caries Frequency. *American Journal of Physical Anthropology*, Vol. 108, No.2, (June 1999), pp. 237-240, ISSN 1096-8644

Esclassan, R.; Grimoud, A.M.; Ruas, M.P.; Donat, R.; Sevin, A.; Astie, F.; Lucas, S. & Crubézy, E. (2009). Dental caries, tooth wear and diet in an adult medieval (12-14th century) population from mediterranean France. *Archives of Oral Biology*, Vol.54, No.3, (March 2009), pp. 287-297, ISSN 0003-9969

Espeland, M.A.; Murphy, W.C. & Leverett, D.H. (1988). Assessing diagnostic reliability and estimating incidence rates associated with a strictly progressive disease: Dental caries. *Statistics in Medicine*, Vol.7, No.3, (March 1988), pp. 403–416, ISSN 1097-0258

Fitzgerald, C.M. & Saunders, S.R. (2005). Test of Histological Methods of Determining Chronology of Accentuated Striae in Deciduous Teeth. *American Journal of Physical Anthropology*, Vol.127, No.3, (July 2005), pp. 277-290, ISSN 1096-8644

Garcin, V.; Velemínský, P.; Trefný, P.; Alduc-Le Bagousse, A.; Lefebvre, A. & Bruzek, J. (2010). Dental health and lifestyle in four early mediaeval juvenile populations: Comparisons between urban and rural individuals, and between coastal and inland settlements. *Homo*, Vol.61, No.6, (December 2010), pp. 421-439, ISSN 0018-442X

Gibbons, R.J. & van Houte, J. (1975). Dental Caries. *Annual Revue of Medicine*, Vol.26, No.2, (February 1975), pp. 121-136, ISSN 0066-4219

Goodman, A.H. & Armelagos, G.J. (1985). Factors Affecting the Distribution of Enamel Hypoplasias Within the Human Permanent Dentition. *American Journal of Physical Anthropology*, Vol.68, No.4, (December 1985), pp. 479-493, ISSN 1096-8644

Goodman, A.H.; Pelto, G.H. & Allen, L.H. (1988). Socioeconomic and nutritional status correlates of enamel developmental defects in mild-to moderately malnourished Mexican children. *American Journal of Physical Anthropology*, Vol.75, No.2, (February 1988), pp. 215, ISSN 1096-8644

Greksa, L.P.; Rie, N.; Islam, A.R.; Maki, U. & Omori, K. (2007). Growth and Health Status of Street Children in Dhaka, Bangladesh. *American Journal of Human Biology*, Vol.19, No.1, (January-February 2007), pp.51-60, ISSN 1520-6300

Halcrow, S.E. & Tayles, N. (2008). The Bioarchaeological Investigation of Childhood and Social Age: Problems and Prospects. *Journal of Archaeological Method and Theory*, Vol.15, No.2, (June 2008), pp. 190-215, ISSN 1573-7764

Hauser, R.M. (1994). Measuring Socioeconomic Status in Studies of Child Development. *Child Development*, Vol.65, No.6, (December 1994), pp.1541-1545, ISSN 1467-8624

Havelkova, P.; Villote, S.; Velemínský, P.; Poláček, L. & Dobisikova, M. (2011). Enthesopathies and Activity Patterns in the Early Medieval Greater Moravian Population (9.-10. century AD): Evidence of Division of Labour. *International Journal of Osteoarchaeology*, Vol.21, No.4, (July-August 2011), pp. 487-504, ISSN 1099-1212

Henneberg, M.; Brush, G. & Harrison, G.A. (2001). Growth of Specific Muscle Strength Between 6 and 18 Years in Contrasting Socioeconomic Conditions. *American Journal of Physical Anthropology*, Vol.115, No.1, (May 2001), pp. 62-70, ISSN 1096-8644

Herold, M. (2008). *Sex differences in mortality in lower Austria and Vienna in the early medieval period: an investigation and evaluation of possible contributing factors*. Ph.D. Thesis dissertation, University of Vienna, Vienna, Austria

Heuzé, Y. & Cardoso, H.F.V. (2008). Testing the Quality of Nonadult Bayesian Dental Age Assessment Methods to Juvenile Skeletal Remains: The Lisbon Collection Children and Secular Trend Effects. *American Journal of Physical Anthropology*, Vol.135, No.3, (March 2008), pp. 275-283, ISSN 1096-8644

Hillson, S. (1979). Diet and dental disease. *World Archaeology*, Vol.11, No.2, (March 1979), pp. 147-162, ISSN 1470-1375

Hillson, S. (1992). Impression and replica methods for studying hypoplasia and perikymata on human tooth crown surfaces from archaeological sites. *International Journal of Osteoarchaeology*, Vol.2, No.1, (March 1992), pp. 65–78, ISSN 1099-1212

Hillson, S. (2001). Recording Dental Caries in Archaeological Human Remains. *International Journal of Osteoarchaeology*, Vol.11, No.4, (July-August 2001), pp. 249-289, ISSN 1099-1212

Hillson, S. & Bond, S. (1997). Relationship of Enamel Hypoplasia to the Pattern of Tooth Crown Growth: A Discussion. *American Journal of Physical Anthropology*, Vol.104, No.1, (September 1997), pp. 89-103, ISSN 1096-8644

Humphrey, L.T. & King, T. (2000). Childhood stress: A lifetime legacy. *Anthropologie*, Vol. 38, No.1, (January-July 2002), pp. 33-49, ISNN 0323–1119

Johansson, I.; Larsson, B.; Nordlund, A. & Ericson, T. (1994). Diet and dental caries. *American Journal of Clinical Nutrition*, Vol.59, No.4, (April 1994), pp. 788S, ISSN 1938-3207

Khan, F.; Young, W.G.; Shahabi, S. & Daley, T.J. (1999). Dental cervical lesions associated with occlusal erosion and attrition. *Australian Dental Journal*, Vol.44, No.3, (September 1999), pp. 176-186, ISSN 1834-7819

Kim, J. & Durden, E. (2007). Socioeconomic status and age trajectories of health. *Social Science & Medicine*, Vol.65, No.12, (December 2007), pp. 2489-2502, ISSN 0277-9536

Klanica, Z. (2006a). *Nechvalin, Prusanky. Vier slawische Nekropolen. Teil I.*, Archäologisches Institut Der Akademie der Wissenschaften der Tschechischen Republik, ISBN 80-86023-75-3, Brno, Czech Republic

Klanica, Z. (2006b.) *Nechvalin, Prusanky. Vier slawische Nekropolen. Teil II.*, Archäologisches Institut Der Akademie der Wissenschaften der Tschechischen Republik, ISBN 80-86023-75-3, Brno, Czech Republic

Klein, H. & Palmer, C.E. (1941). Studies on Dental Caries. XII. Comparisons of the Caries Susceptibility of the Various Morphological Types of Permanent Teeth. *Journal of Dental Research*, Vol.20, No.3, (June 1941), pp. 203-216, ISSN 1544-0591

König, K.G. & Navia, J.M. (1995). Nutritional role of sugars in oral health. *American Journal of Clinical Nutrition*, Vol.62, No.1, (July 1995), pp. 275S-283S, ISSN 1938-3207

Landis, J.R. & Koch, G.G. (1977). The Measurment of Observer Agreement for Categorical Data. *Biometrics*, Vol.33, No2, (June 1977), pp. 159-174, ISSN 1541-0420

Leger, L. (1868). *Cyrille et Méthode: étude historique sur la conversion des slaves au christianisme*. A. Franck, Paris, France.

Lewis, M.E. (2007). *The Bioarchaeology of Children. Perspectives from Biological and Forensic Anthropology*. Cambridge University Press, ISBN 052-1836-02-6, Cambridge, United Kingdom

Lewis, M.E. & Gowland, R.L. (2007). Brief and Precarious Lives: Infant Mortality in
    Contrasting Sites from Medieval and Post-Medieval England (AD 850-1859).
    American Journal of Physical Anthropology, Vol.134, No.1, (September 2007), pp. 117-
    129, ISSN 1096-8644

Li, Y. & Wang, W. (2002). Predicting Caries in PermanentTeeth from Caries in Primary
    Teeth: An Eight-year Cohort Study. *Journal of Dental Research*, Vol.81, No.8, (August
    2002), pp. 561-566, ISSN 1544-0591

Lukacs, J.R. (1995). The 'Caries Correction Factor': a New Method of Calibrating Dental
    Caries Rates to Compensate for Antemortem Loss of Teeth. *International Journal of
    Osteoarchaeology*, Vol.5, No.2, (June 1995), pp.151-156, ISSN 1099-1212

Lukacs, J.R. (1999a). Enamel Hypoplasia in Deciduous Teeth of Great Apes: Do Differences
    in Defect Prevalence Imply Differential Levels of Physiological Stress? *American
    Journal of Physical Anthropology*, Vol.110, No.3, (November 1999), pp.351-363, ISSN
    1096-8644

Lukacs, J.R. (1999b). Interproximal Contact Hypoplasia in Primary Teeth: A New Enamel
    Defect With Anthropological and Clinical Relevance. *American Journal of Human
    Biology*, Vol.11, No.6, (November-December 1999), pp. 718-734, ISSN 1520-6300

Lukacs, J.R. (2001). Enamel Hypoplasia in the Deciduous Teeth of Great Apes: Variation in
    Prevalence and Timing of Defects. *American Journal of Physical Anthropology*,
    Vol.116, No.3, (November 2001), pp. 199-208, ISSN 1096-8644

Lukacs, J.R.; Nelson, G.C. & Walimbe, S.R. (2001a). Enamel Hypoplasia and Childhood
    Stress in Prehistory: New Data from India and Southwest Asia. *Journal of
    Archaeological Science*, Vol.28, No.11, (November 2001), pp. 1159-1169, ISSN 0305-
    4403

Lukacs, J.R.; Walimbe, S.R. & Floyd, B. (2001b). Epidemiology of Enamel Hypoplasia in
    Deciduous Teeth: Explaining Variation in Prevalence in Western India. *American
    Journal of Human Biology*, Vol.13, No.6, (November-December 2001), pp. 788-807,
    ISSN 1520-6300

Moorrees, C.F.A.; Fanning, E.A. & Hunt, E.E. (1963a). Age Variation of Formation Stages for
    Ten Permanent Teeth. *Journal of Dental Research*, Vol.42, No.6, (November 1963),
    pp.1490-1502, ISSN 1544-0591

Moorrees, C.F.A.; Fanning, E.A. & Hunt, E.E. (1963b). Formation and Resorption of three
    Deciduous Teeth in Children. *American Journal of Physical Anthropology*, Vol.21,
    No.2, (June 1963), pp. 205-213, ISSN 1096-8644

Navia, J.M. (1994). Carbohydrates and dental health. *American Journal of Clinical Nutrition*,
    Vol.59, No.3, (March 1994), pp.719S-727S, ISSN 1938-3207

Norén, J.G. (1983). Enamel structure in deciduous teeth from low-birth-weight infants. *Acta
    Odontologica Scandinavica*, Vol.41, No.6, (January 1983), pp. 355-362, ISSN 1502-3850

O'Sullivan, D.M. & Tinanoff, N. (1993). Maxillary Anterior Caries Associated with Increased
    Caries Risk in Other Primary Teeth. *Journal of Dental Research*, Vol.72, No.12,
    (December 1993), pp. 1577-1580, ISSN 1544-0591

O'Sullivan, E.A.; Williams, S.A. & Curzon, M.E. (1992). Dental Caries in Relation to
    Nutritional Stress in Early English Child Populations. *Pediatric Dentistry*, Vol.14,
    No.1, (January-February), pp. 26-29, ISSN 0164-1263

Obertová, Z. (2005). Environmental stress in the Early Mediaeval Slavic population at Borovce
    (Slovakia). *Homo*, Vol.55, No.3, (February 2005), pp. 283-291, ISSN 0018-442X

Obertová, Z. & Thurzo, M. (2008). Relationship between Cribra Orbitalia and Enamel Hypoplasia in the Early Medieval Slavic Population at Borovce, Slovakia. *International Journal of Osteoarchaeology*, Vol.18, No.3, (May-June 2008), pp. 280-292, ISSN 1099-1212

Ogden, A.R.; Pinhasi, R. & White, W.J. (2007). Gross Enamel Hypoplasia in Molars From Subadults in a 16th-18th Century London Graveyard. *American Journal of Physical Anthropology*, Vol.133, No.3, (July 2007), pp. 957-966, ISSN 1096-8644

Oyamada, J.; Igawa, K.; Kitagawa, Y.; Manabe, Y.; Kato, K.; Matsushita, T. & Rokutanda, A. (2008). Pathology of deciduous teeth in the samurai and commoner children of early modern Japan. *Anthropological Science*, Vol.116, No.1, (January 2008), pp. 9-15, ISSN 1348-8570

Palubeckaité, Z.; Jankauskas, R. & Boldsen, J.L. (2002). Enamel Hypoplasia in Danish and Lithuanian Late Medieval / Early Modern Samples: A Possible Reflection of Child Morbidity and Mortality Patterns. *International Journal of Osteoarchaeology*, Vol.12, No.3, (May-June 2002), pp. 189-201, ISSN 1099-1212

Pinhasi, R.; Teschler-Nicola, M.; Knaus, A. & Shaw, P. (2005). Cross-Population Analysis of the Growth of Long Bones and the Os Coxae of Three Early Medieval Austrian Populations. *American Journal of Human Biology*, Vol.17, No.4, (July-August 2005), pp. 470-488, ISSN 1520-6300

Poláček, L. (2000). *Tereni vyzkum v Mikulcicich (Mikulcice - pruvodce, svazek 1)*, AU AV CR, ISBN 80-86023-26-5, Brno, Czech Republic

Poláček, L. (2008). Great Moravia, the Power Centre at Mikulcice and the Issue of the Socio-economic Stucture. In: *Studien zum Burgwall von Mikulcice VIII*, P. Velemínský & L. Poláček, (Eds.), 11-44, Archäologisches Institut Der Akademie der Wissenschaften der Tschechischen Republik, ISBN 978-80-86023-74-8, Brno, Czech Republic

Poláček, L. & Marek, O. (2005). Grundlager der Topographie des Burgwalls von Mikulčice. Die Grabungsflächen 1954-1992. In: *Studien zum Burgwall von Mikulčice VII*, L. Poláček, (Ed.), 9-358, Archäologisches Institut Der Akademie der Wissenschaften der Tschechischen Republik, ISBN 808-6023-57-5, Brno, Czech Republic

Poláček, L.; Mazuch, M. & Baxa, P. (2006). Mikulčice-Kopčany. Stav a perspektivy výzkumu. *Archeologické rozhledy*, Vol.58, No.4, (October 2006), pp. 623-642, ISSN 0323-1267

Reich, E.; Lussi, A. & Newbrun, E. (1999). Caries-risk assessment. *International Dental Journal*, Vol.49, No.1, (February 1999), pp.15-26, ISSN 0020-6539

Reid, D.J. & Dean, M.C. (2000). Brief Communication: The Timing of Linear Hypoplasias on Human Anterior Teeth. *American Journal of Physical Anthropology*, Vol.113, No.1, (September 2000), pp.135-139, ISSN 1096-8644

Ritz-Timme, S.; Cattaneo, C.; Collins, M.J.; Waite, E.R.; Schütz, H.W.; Kaatsch, H-J. & Borrman, H.I.M. (2000). Ages estimation: The state of the art in relation to the specific demands of forensic practise. *International Journal of Legal Medecine*, Vol.113, No.3, (May 2000), pp. 129-136, ISSN 1437-1596

Ritzman, T.B.; Baker, B.J. & Schwartz, G.T. (2008). A Fine Line: A Comparison of Methods for Estimating Ages of Linear Enamel Hypoplasia Formation. *American Journal of Physical Anthropology*, Vol.135, No.3, (March 2008), pp. 348-361, ISSN 1096-8644

Riva, M.; Curtis, S.; Gauvin, L. & Fagg, J. (2009). Unravelling the extent of inequalities in health accross urban and rural areas: Evidence from a national sample in England. *Social Science & Medicine*, Vol.68, No.4, (February 2009), pp. 654-663, ISSN 0277-9536

Rudney, J.D.; Katz, R.V. & Brand, J.W. (1983). Interobserver reliability of methods for paleopathological diagnosis of dental caries. *American Journal of Physical Anthropology*, Vol.62, No.2, (June 1983), pp. 243–248, ISSN 1096-8644

Saunders, S.R.; De Vito, C. & Katzenberg, M.A. (1997). Dental Caries in Nineteenth Century Upper Canada. *American Journal of Physical Anthropology*, Vol.104, No.1, (September 1997), pp. 71-87, ISSN 1096-8644

Saunders, S.R. & Hoppa, R.D. (1993). Growth Deficit in Survivors and Non-Survivors: Biological Mortality Bias in Subadult Skeletal Samples. *Yearbook of Physical Anthropology*, Vol.36, No. Supplement 17, pp.127-151, ISSN 1096-8644

Saunders, S.R.; Hoppa, R.D.; Macchiarelli, R. & Bondioli, L. (2000). Investigating variability in human dental development in the past. *Anthropologie*, Vol.38, No.1, (January-July 2002), pp. 101-107, ISNN 0323-1119

Scheuer, L. & Black, S. (2000a). Development and ageing of the juvenile skeleton, In: *Human osteology in archaeology and forensic medicine*, M. Cox & S. Mays, (Eds.), 9-21, Greenwich Medical Media, ISBN 978-184-1100-46-3, London, United Kingdom

Scheuer, L. & Black, S. (2000b). *Developmental Juvenile Osteology*. Elsevier Academic Press, ISBN 0-12-624000-0, London, United Kingdom

Schmitt, A. (2005). Une nouvelle méthode pour estimer l'âge au décès des adultes à partir de la surface sacro-pelvienne iliaque, *Bulletins et Mémoires de la Société d'Anthropologie de Paris*, Vol.17, No.1-2, (January-July 2005), pp. 89-101, ISSN 0037-8984

Schneider, K.N. (1986). Dental Caries, Enamel Composition, and Subsistence Among Prehistoric Amerindians of Ohio. *American Journal of Physical Anthropology*, Vol.71, No.1, (September 1986), pp. 95-102, ISSN 1096-8644

Skinner, M.F. & Goodman, A.H. (1992). Anthropological Uses of Developmental Defects of Enamel, In: *Skeletal Biology of Past Peoples: Reasearch Methods*, S.R. Saunders & M.A. Katzenberg, (Eds.), 153-174, Wiley-Liss, ISBN 978-047-1561-38-5, New York, United States

Skinner, M.F. & Hung, J.T.W. (1989). Social and Biological Correlates of Localized Enamel Hypoplasia of the Human Deciduous Canine Tooth. *American Journal of Physical Anthropology*, Vol.79, No.2, (June 1989), pp. 159-175, ISSN 1096-8644

Šlaus, M.; Kollmann, D.; Novak, S.A. & Novak, M. (2002). Temporal trends in demographic profiles and stress levels in medieval (6th-13th centuries) population samples from continental Croatia. *Croatian Medical Journal*, Vol.43, No.5, (October 2002), pp. 598–605, ISSN 1332-8166

Stloukal, M. (1967). Druhé pohřebiště na hradišti „Valy" u Mikulčic. *Památky archeologické*, Vol.58, No.1, (January 1967), pp. 272-319, ISSN 0031-0506

Sweeney, E.A.; Cabrera, J.; Urrutia, J. & Mata, L. (1969). Factors Associated with Linear Hypoplasia of Human Deciduous Incisors. *Journal of Dental Research*, Vol.48, No.6, (November 1969), pp. 1275-1279, ISSN 1544-0591

Sweeney, E.A.; Saffir, A.J. & De Leon, R. (1971). Linear hypoplasia of deciduous incisor teeth in malnourished children. *American Journal of Clinical Nutrition*, Vol.24, No.1, (January 1971), pp. 29-31, ISSN 0002-9165

Taji, S.; Hughes, T.; Rogers, J. & Townsend, G. (2000). Localised enamel hypoplasia of human deciduous canines: genotype or environment? *Australian Dental Journal*, Vol.45, No.2, (June 2000), pp. 83-90, ISSN 1834-7819

Třeštík, D. (2001). *Vznik Velké Moravy. Moravané, Cechové a Stredni Evropa v Letech 791-871,* Nakladatelstvi Lidové Noviny, ISBN 807-1066-46-X, Prague, Czech Republic

Ubelaker, D.H. (1978). *Human Skeletal Remains: Excavation, Analysis and Interpretation,* Smithsonian Institute Press, ISBN 978-020-2362-39-7, Washington, United States

Ulijaszek, S.J. & Lourie, J.A. (1997). Anthropometry in Health Assessment: The Importance of Measurement Error. *Collegium Anthropologicum,* Vol.21, No.2, (July 1997), pp. 429-438, ISSN 0350-6134

Van de Poel, E.; O'Donnell, O. & Van Doorslaer, E. (2007). Are urban children really healthier ? Evidence from 47 developing countries. *Social Science & Medicine,* Vol.65, No.10, (November 2007), pp. 1986-2003, ISSN 0277-9536

Velemínský, P. (2000). *Mikulčice-Kostelisko. Nekteré kostni projevy nespecifické zateze a moznosti stanoveni pokrevne pribuzenskych vztahu na zaklade morfologické podobnosti.* Ph.D. Thesis Dissertation, Charles University, Prague, Czech Republic

Velemínský, P.; Likovský, J.; Trefný, P.; Dobisíková, M.; Velemínská, J.; Poláček, L. & Hanáková, H. (2005) Großmährisches Gräberfeld auf „Kostelisko" im Suburbium des Mikulčicer Burgwalls. Demographie, Spuren nicht spezifischer Belastung physiologischen und physischen Charakters auf Skeletten, Gesundheitszustand, In: *Studien zum Burgwall von Mikulčice, Band VI,* L. Poláček, (Ed.), 539-633, Archäologisches Institut Der Akademie der Wissenschaften der Tschechischen Republik, ISBN 808-6023-31-1, Brno, Czech Republic

Vodanović, M.; Brkić, H.; Šlaus, M. & Demo, Z. (2005). The frequency and distribution of caries in the mediaeval population of Bijelo Brdo in Croatia (10th-11th century). *Archives of Oral Biology,* Vol.50, No.7, (July 2005), pp. 669-680, ISSN 0003-9969

Walker, P.L. & Hewlett, B.S. (1990). Dental Health Diet and Social Status among Central African Foragers and Farmers. *American Anthropologist,* Vol.92, No.2, (June 1990), pp. 383-398, ISSN 1548-1433

Watt, M.E.; Lunt, D.A. & Gilmour, W.H. (1997). Caries prevalence in the deciduous dentition of a mediaeval population from the southwest of Scotland. *Archives of Oral Biology,* Vol.42, No.12, (December 1997), pp. 811–820, ISSN 0003-9969

Williams, S.A. & Curzon, M.E.J. (1985). Dental caries in a Scottish medieval child population. *Caries Research,* Vol.19, No. 2, (March 1985), pp. 162, ISSN 0008-6568

Williams, N. & Galley, C. (1995). Urban-rural Differentials in Infant Mortality in Victorian England. *Population Studies,* Vol.49, No.3, (September 1995), pp. 401-420, ISSN 1477-4747

Wood, J.W.; Milner, G.R.; Harpending, H.C. & Weiss, K.M. (1992). The Osteological Paradox. Problems of Inferring Prehistoric Health from Skeletal Samples. *Current Anthropology,* Vol.33, No.4, (August-October 1992), pp. 343-370, ISSN 0011-3204

Wright, L.E. (1997). Intertooth Patterns of Hypoplasia Expression: Implications for Childhood Health in the Classic Maya Collapse. *American Journal of Physical Anthropology,* Vol.102, No.2, (February 1997), pp.233-247, ISSN 1096-8644

Wright, L.E. & Yoder, C.J. (2003). Recent progess in bioarchaeology: Approaches to the osteological paradox. *Journal of Archaeological Research,* Vol.11, No.1, (March 2003), pp. 43-70, ISSN 1573-7756

Internet site of the World Heritage Center of Unesco: http://whc.unesco.org

4

Susceptibility of Enamel Treated with Bleaching Agents to Mineral Loss After Cariogenic Challenge

Hüseyin Tezel and Hande Kemaloğlu
Ege University, Faculty of Dentistry,
Department of Restorative Dentistry and Endodontics, Izmir,
Turkey

1. Introduction

As patients and consumers demand not only a healthy mouth but also a perfect appearance, vital bleaching of teeth has gained interest. It has been accepted as one the most effective methods of treating discolored teeth and considered to be a conservative approach towards obtaining esthetic or cosmetic results rather than other methods such as veneering or crowning. Procedures that utilize different concentrations of carbamide peroxide (CP) or hydrogen peroxide (HP) have been commonly used by dentists as "in office" or by patients as "home bleaching" applications. Other than these, over the counter products have been widely used by patients; however they cannot be considered as one of the "bleaching treatments".

The efficacy of bleaching is influenced by many factors like the type, concentration of the bleaching agent, time it is applied, application method used (heat, light, laser, etc.) cause of the stain and the condition of teeth. Procedures apparently rely on an extended period of contact between the bleaching agent and the teeth to accomplish the bleaching. The decomposition of hydrogen peroxide results in oxygen and per-hydroxyl free radicals that oxidize the stained macromolecules and break them down into smaller lighter colored fragments. Then the fragments diffuse across the tooth surface resulting in the bleaching effect (Haywood, 1992; Chen et al., 1993). The oxidation reaction should not exceed the saturation point in which the organic and inorganic elements of enamel and dentin are damaged. Otherwise, the crystals of mine matrix proteins lead to adverse changes in the morphology of the tooth surface and weakened structure (Haywood & Heymann, 1989; Goldstein&Garber, 1995). Studies (Seghi RR&Denry, 1992; Justino et al., 2004; Flaitz & Hicks, 1996; Spalding et al., 2003; Türkun et al., 2002; Bitter, 1992; Lopes et al., 2002; Hegedüs et al.,1999; Rotstein et al.,1996; Potocnick et al., 2000; Tezel et al., 2007.) have shown that bleaching agents can cause structural alterations on enamel surface and that the biomechanical properties of the enamel can change. In addition Basting and others (Basting et al., 2001) reported the possibility of formatting of active caries lesions after bleaching process since they diffuse through the enamel by demineralization.

2. Effects of bleaching agents on enamel surface

Calcium and phosphorus are present in the hydroxyapatite crystals, the main building block of dental hard tissue. Changes in Ca/P ratio indicate alterations in the inorganic components of hydroxyapatite. In the previous studies it has been shown that the bleaching agents cause calcium loss in hard dental tissues, change Ca/P ratio and surface alterations depending on their concentration. The linear relationship between decrease in enamel hardness and Ca^{2+} and PO_4^{3-} loss shows that hardness measurements can be used as an indication of the degree of enamel mineralization which relates to enamel caries. Ingram and Ferjerskov (Ingram & Ferjerskov, 1986) observed that macroscopically the degree of chemical attack roughly correlated with the appearance of discrete white spot lesions where approximately 7 µg or more calcium had been removed from the experimental area (1.77 mm²). This means that when approximately 3.95 µg of calcium loss is observed in a surface of mm², the surface cannot be remineralized.

Additionally, *in vitro* studies have shown a close correlation between the bleaching agent effects and the enamel surface changes (Zalkind et al., 1996; Titley et al., 1988). There are also some reports that bleaching agents promote chemical and microstructural changes in enamel similar to initial caries lesions but it has been noted that these alterations have no clinical significance. Demineralization process begins with the loss of calcium ions from the surface apatite crystals that form the bulk of three calcified dental tissues. Under normal circumstances, this loss of calcium (demineralization) is compensated by the uptake of calcium (remineralization) from tooth's microenvironment. This dynamic process of demineralization and remineralization take place more or less continually and equally in a favorable oral environment. In an unfavorable environment, the remineralization rate does not sufficiently neutralize the rate of demineralization, and thus caries occurs (Davidson et al., 1973). It has been reported that most of the bleaching agents caused changes in the levels of calcium phosphorus, sulfur and potassium in dental tissues and that bleaching agents may have a possible influence on active caries lesions in enamel and dentin (Rotstein et al.,1996; Basting et al., 2001). It is still a question whether the enamel would be more susceptible to cariogenic challenge after the bleaching process. Little is known about this issue. The controversial results of existing reports and the continuous appearance of new bleaching products that are on the market demand more research in this field.

This is particularly evident in a study demonstrated by *Tezel et al* (Tezel et al., 2007) who showed different amounts of Ca^{2+} loss from enamel surface after bleaching with three different concentrations of bleaching agents. Premolar teeth were divided into four pieces and each piece was bleached with one of the bleaching agents (38% HP, 35% HP with light and 10% CP) leaving one as a control. Then the specimens were covered with wax as to expose a round window area on 6.83 mm² and immersed in an artificial caries solution of acetic acid buffered with 0.34 M sodium acetate (pH=4). The buffer solution was refreshed every four days till the 16th day. The previous solutions were kept to be tested afterwards for their Ca^{2+} loss with atomic absorption spectrometer (AAS). The loss of Ca^{2+} in the groups 38% HP, 35% HP with light activation, 10% CP and the control were evaluated cumulatively every four days and at the end of the 16th day, 27.52±5.22 µg/ml, 25.15±4.99 µg/ml, 19.53±4.03 µg/ml and 18.35±4.00 µg/ml were obtained in total, respectively (Table 1, Fig. 1).

	N		Days 1-4	Days 5-8	Days 9-12	Days 13-16	Total
38% HP	10	Mean	5.22	4.91	6.46	10.93	27.52
		Std Dev	1.78	1.02	2.43	2.96	5.22
		Min.	1.37	3.23	2.81	5.54	20.88
		Max.	6.97	6.34	11.02	14.67	38.09
35% HP	10	Mean	5.72	4.42	6.27	8.74	25.15
		Std Dev	1.41	0.90	2.01	4.98	4.99
		Min.	3.86	3.23	2.81	3.72	19.13
		Max.	8.21	6.34	10.11	19.23	34.98
10% CP	10	Mean	4.10	3.61	4.17	7.64	19.53
		Std Dev	1.69	1.90	1.51	3.55	4.03
		Min.	1.99	1.37	1.89	4.63	14.20
		Max.	3.73	6.84	4.56	10.04	12.57
Control Group	10	Mean	3.48	3.42	3.89	7.55	18.35
		Std Dev	1.32	1.38	1.34	1.96	4.00
		Min.	1.37	1.37	1.89	4.63	12.76
		Max.	5.72	6.34	6.46	11.02	25.56

Table 1. Release of calcium (Ca^{2+}) from the specimens after treatment with bleaching agents in mm^2 ($\mu g/ml$).

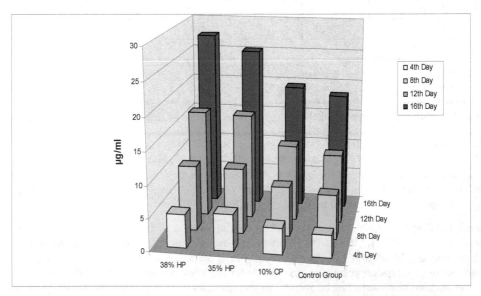

Fig. 1. Release of Ca^{2+} from the specimens to the buffer solution after treatment with bleaching agents on the 4th, 8th, 12th and 16th days cumulatively ($\mu g/ml$).

According to the statistical analysis, all the bleaching agents increased the Ca^{2+} in the solutions and all the agents other than CP were statistically different from the control group. And starting from the fourth day, the amount of Ca^{2+} release varied for the control and test groups. These differences are considered to be due to the variety of concentrations of the bleaching agents which were applied to the enamel. When 38% and light activated 35% HP groups were compared to the control group, it was observed that the difference Ca^{2+} loss was statistically significant and the high concentration of HP agents changed the surface morphology of the enamel. Thus, the resistance of enamel surfaces decreased in these groups when there was an acid attack. The use of HP or CP as bleaching agents reportedly decreased the Ca/P ratio on the enamel surface. It should also be mentioned that, HP was the only material that significantly reduced the Ca/P ratio in all these tissues. Most of the bleaching agents examined, caused changes of calcium, phosphorous, sulfur and potassium in the tissues. It was important to examine the effects of the oxidation agents on all the dental hard tissues because contact could occur during internal and/or external bleaching procedures, or they could inadvertently come into contact with dentin in carious lesions, enamel defects or abrasions.

In the group to which 10% CP was applied, a difference of Ca^{2+} loss was observed when it was compared to the control group after the 16th day, but this difference was not statistically significant (Table 2).

Materials	Days 1-4	Days 5-8	Days 9-12	Days 13-16	Total
38% HP X 35% HP	-	-	-	-	-
38% HP X 10% CP	-	*	*	*	*
38% HP X Control	*	*	*	*	*
35% HP X 10%CP	*	-	*	-	*
35% HP X Control	*	-	*	-	*
10% CP X Control	-	-	-	-	-
* Statistically significant differences between the groups (p<.05) - No statistically significant differences (p>.05)					

Table 2. Statistical differences of the test groups in the end of the 4th, 8th, 12th and 16th days.

The reason why there occurred a close demineralization to the control group was due to low HP concentration of 10% CP. In accordance with this study, Haywood et al (Haywood et al., 1990) reported no change in the surface morphology of the enamel with 10% CP, whereas, McGuckin et al (McGucking et al., 1992), Bitter & Sanders (Bitter & Sanders, 1993) observed slight surface modifications of teeth treated with 10% CP.

Tezel et al (Tezel et al., 2007) also examined that there was a sudden rise of Ca^{2+} discharge on the 16th day (Table 1). When they compared the results, they have observed that Ca^{2+} releases on the 4th, 8th and 12th days were similar (Fig 1). The data had been measured twice with atomic absorption spectrophotometer, and the same results were obtained each time. So the sudden rise could not be related to the inaccuracy of the measurements. Thus, they have assumed that the organo-inorganic structure of enamel got weaker by the 12th day, reaching a critical point on the 16th day when sudden Ca^{2+} discharge had been observed.

In addition, it has been shown that the control and CP are similar in demineralization and HP is so different. The 10% CP disassociates into 3% HP and approximately 7% urea. The HP further degrades into oxygen and water, while the urea degrades into ammonia and carbon dioxide. The ammonia and carbon dioxide elevate the pH. Hence, a CP solution will supply urea and may raise the pH of solution when used clinically. In addition it was pointed out that after 15 minutes of treatment with CP the pH of saliva increases to greater than baseline because of chemical reactions to neutralization of acidic CP by saliva

Tezel *et al* (Tezel et al., 2007) claimed that the Ca^{2+} loss as a result of bleaching process can be named as "erosion" since the erosion is defined as "the physical result of a pathologic, chronic and localized loss of dental hard tissue which is chemically etched away from tooth surface by acid and/or chelation without bacterial involvement" (Imfeld, 1996). However it should also be mentioned that with in the presence of dental plaque, the outcomes could be very different.

There are published studies showing that the bleaching treatments can cause loss of mineral content which may widen the space between the enamel prisms. This can influence caries activity in cooperation with the increased surface roughness and gingival plaque formation (Flaitz et al.,1996; Quirynen&Bollen, 1995; Perdigao et al., 1998). As a result, *Streptococcus mutans* adhesion is included in the action which might be related to caries formation if undesirable conditions continue to develop (Hosaya et al, 2003).

Many researchers have reported the effects of different bleaching agents to dental hard tissues. Lewinstein *et al* (Lewinstein et al, 1994) pointed out that the microhardness of bleached enamel is decreased after bleaching with hydrogen peroxide and some have reported that there are no changes in the microhardness values of enamel when treated with 10% CP (Potocnick et al., 2000; Murchinson et al., 1992; Seghi&Denhy, 1992). There are also some studies which reported a decrease in microhardess values after application of these bleaching agents (Attin et al,1997; Smidt et al.,1998; Rodrigues et al., 2001). It can be concluded that most of the bleaching agents cause alterations on the enamel surface and decrease in microhardness some causing groves on the surface and even effect the inner surface (Hegedüs et al.,1999; Rodrigues et al., 2001).

The decomposition of HP results in oxygen and per-hydroxyl free radicals, which then oxidize the stained macromolecules and break them down into smaller fragments. Then the fragments diffuse across the tooth surface, resulting in the bleaching effect. To accelerate this reaction light sources such as blue halogen light, light-emitting diode (LED)-laser system, blue plasma arc lamp, argon laser, GAAlAs diode laser, ultraviolet light, ER:YAG laser and CO_2 laser are used (Sydney et al.,2002; Wetter et al., 2004; Zhang et al., 2007) But today, lights and lasers are the preferred activation methods. The use of activation methods has shortened the extensive period of time, which involves the direct contact of the high concentrated bleaching agents with the tooth surface that may cause a certain amount of enamel matrix degradation. A shortened treatment period may eradicate the side effects of high concentrated HP.

Tezel *et al* conducted an *in vitro* study (Tezel et al., 2011) aiming to compare the Ca^{2+} loss after activating the bleaching agents with halogen light and diode laser. The specimens were prepared with the same method of their earlier study. The bleaching agents (38% HP with halogen light activation, 38% HP with diode laser activation, and 10% CP) were applied according to manufacturers' instructions. Then the same artificial caries formation method was used. However this time in the study, inductively coupled plasma mass spectrometry

(ICP-MS) was used to measure the calcium ions released, which is a very precise method that can determine the very low concentrations of ions. When the results were examined, the Ca^{2+} ions released from CP group (12.88 µg/ml) was very close to the control group (11.97µg/ml) and there was no statistical difference between them (p>0.05). The highest value was obtained from the 38% HP group with light activation (16.20 µg/ml) and this result was statistically higher than the other groups (p<0.05). Laser activated group (14.10 µg/ml) did not show any statistically different result than the CP group (p>0.05). However; it was statistically different than the control group (p<0.05) (Table 3, 4 and Fig. 2).

		Days 1-4	Days 5-8	Days 9-12	Days 13-16	Total
10% CP	Mean	3.03	3.28	3.30	3.26	12.88
	Std Dev	0.42	0.58	0.48	0.30	1.48
	Min.	2.55	2.60	2.83	2.80	11.04
	Max.	4.06	4.47	4.16	3.84	14.59
38% HP with light	Mean	3.66	4.19	4.24	4.10	16.20
	Std Dev	0.70	0.44	0.49	0.37	1.67
	Min.	2.54	3.58	3.66	3.69	13.79
	Max.	5.24	5.03	5.10	5.00	19.28
38% HP with diode laser	Mean	3.23	3.66	3.65	3.56	14.10
	Std Dev	0.59	0.55	0.66	0.55	2.16
	Min.	2.60	2.68	2.90	2.53	10.71
	Max.	4.52	4.57	4.67	4.47	17.72
Control Group	Mean	2.87	3.06	3.00	3.03	11.97
	Std Dev	0.30	0.43	0.32	0.20	0.87
	Min.	2.52	2.67	2.65	2.81	10.92
	Max.	3.54	3.82	3.69	3.38	13.56

Table 3. Release of Ca^{2+} from the specimens after treatment with bleaching agents (in µg/ml) (n=10 each group).

As mentioned during the study, the bleaching agents were used in accordance with manufacturers' protocols and these were also followed for the activation methods used. The aim was to follow the clinical protocol. According to the manufacturers' instructions, the chemical bleaching without activation is 15 minutes for three times. In total, the contact time for the bleaching gel throughout the study would have been 135 minutes. Activating the bleaching gel with halogen light reduced the contact time to 45 minutes and for the laser activated group to 36 minutes. It can be assumed that the higher concentration of HP could have caused more Ca^{2+} loss than the CP group, but due to laser activation which shortened contact time of the high concentrated bleaching gel, the calcium loss in the laser group was close to the CP group. The results of the study was in correlation with the other *in vitro* bleaching studies that Ca^{2+} loss was lower when lasers were used for the activation of the bleaching agents compared to halogen light.

Materials	Days 1-4	Days 6-8	Days 9-12	Days 13-16	Total
38% HP with light vs. 10% CP	-	*	**	*	*
38% HP with light vs. 38% HP with laser diode	-	-	-	*	*
38% HP with light vs. Control	*	*	**	*	*
38% HP with laser diode vs. 10% CP	-	-	-	-	-
38% HP with laser diode vs. Control	-	-	-	*	*
10% CP vs. Control	-	-	-	-	-
* Statistically significant differences between the groups for Bonferroni test (p<.05). ** Statistically significant differences between the groups for Dunnet C test (p<.05).					

Table 4. Statistical differences of the test groups at end of days 4, 8, 12, and 16.

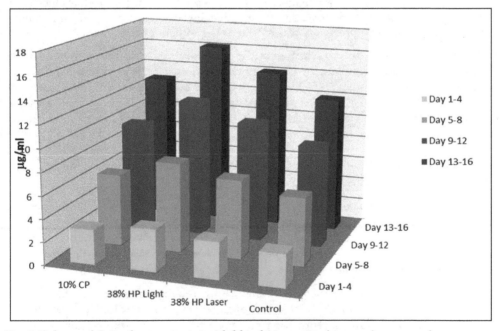

Fig. 2. Release of Ca^{2+} after treatment with bleaching agents (per mm², measured cumulatively).

These mentioned effects of bleaching agents with different concentrations and activation techniques on human enamel surface morphology were observed by Kemaloğlu and Tezel using scanning electron microscopy (SEM; Fei, Quanta Feg 250). The purpose was to compare the changes caused by the bleaching agents visually. Human impacted third molar teeth were rinsed in tap water and were cleaned off plaque and debris with a dental handpiece and brush. The buccal, lingual and occlusal surfaces were checked under a stereomicroscope, and teeth with enamel defects or cracks were rejected. The selected teeth (n=5) were stored in 0.9% saline solution for one week and then rinsed in distilled water. Each tooth was sectioned into five parts, so that five specimens were obtained from each tooth. These specimens were randomly assigned to one of the groups, ensuring that each part of every specimen would be in a different group. Teeth were then covered with wax except for the enamel surface. The groups were as follows:

Group 1 (positive control): No agent was used and they were kept in artificial saliva during the test period.

Group 2 : Treated with 37% orthophosphoric acid (ScotchBond Phosphoric Etchant Kit, 3M ESPE, USA) for 30 seconds.

Group 3: Bleached with 10% carbamide peroxide (CP) (Opalescence PF 10% CP, Ultradent Products Inc, South Jordan, USA) for 8 hours a day, throughout 14 days.

Group 4: Bleached with 38% hydrogen peroxide (HP) (Opalescence Boost 38% HP, Ultradent Products Inc, South Jordan, USA) with light activation for 15 minutes. This procedure was repeated every other day for 3 days.

Group 5: Bleached with 38% HP (Opalescence Boost 38% HP, Ultradent Products Inc, South Jordan, USA) with diode laser activation (LaserSmile, Biolase, USA) in 10 Watt-continuous mode for 12 minutes. This procedure was repeated every other day for 3 days.

Following every session, the bleached teeth were rinsed, dried and topical fluoride agent (Flor-Opal 1.1% NaF, Ultradent Products Inc, South Jordan, USA) was applied for 10 minutes. After the application of the bleaching agents for the prescribed time, the specimens were anticipated in artificial saliva for 12 days to mimic the *in vivo* remineralization condition. Then the specimens were rinsed ultrasonically with water for ten minutes and prepared for scanning electron microscope. After dehydration, enamel surfaces were sputter coated with gold (~ 30-35 nm) and photomicrographs of representative areas were taken at 5000x magnifications. The enamel changes were classified as no alterations, mild or slight alterations and altered surfaces (loss of superficial structure).

A representative SEM image of sound enamel surface stored in artificial saliva (positive control group) is shown in Figure 3. There were no remarkable morphologic alterations on unbleached enamel surfaces. The surface was not completely smooth, however the aprismatic surface layer was uniform. Perikymata was evident all over the surface. In addition, pores could easily be seen and there were some areas that had cracks.

In the second group, the acid-etched samples had a rough and uneven surface, which indicates alterations of the prismatic structure of the enamel due to selective dissolution of the apatite crystals (Figure 4). Formation of an irregular meshwork and dissolution in central (intraprismatic) or peripheral (interprismatic) part of the prism take place as a result of demineralization.

Bleached groups showed alterations on surface smoothness and presented different levels of surface changes. Minor changes of the enamel surface occurred in samples treated with 10% CP for 8 hours daily for 14 days (Figure 5). This aspect suggests a slight increase in the enamel porosity, as compared to the control samples. Mildly changed areas and the noted interprismatic limits are show the surface change.

Mild intraprismatic structure dissolution occured on the surface treated with 38% HP with light activation (Figure 6). The surface alterations were much more significant than the other bleaching groups. Porosity and concavity of the enamel structure increased due to intraprismatic dissolution.

Minor alterations on surface smoothness and mildly increased porosity occurred in the teeth bleached with 38% HP with laser activation (Figure 7). Interprismatic dissolution could clearly be observed. These changes were similar to the image of 10% CP group (Figure 5), but additionally the deposits on the surface were also noted (Figure 7).

Fig. 3. SEM micrograph of the sound enamel surface

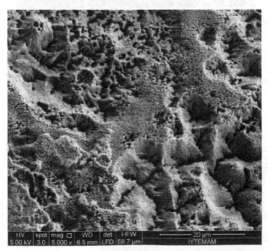

Fig. 4. SEM micrograph of enamel surface treated with 37% orthophosphoric acid

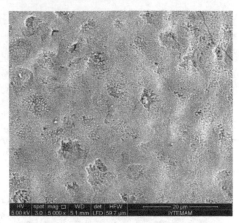

Fig. 5. SEM micrograph of enamel surface treated with 10% CP

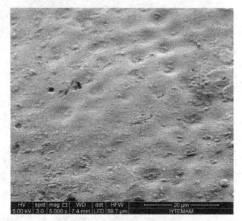

Fig. 6. SEM micrograph of enamel surface treated with 38% HP with light activation

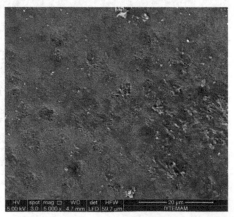

Fig. 7. SEM micrograph of enamel surface treated with 38% HP with diode laser activation

It can be concluded that the Ca^{2+} loss results and surface alterations observed in SEM images were in compliance.

3. Effect of pH values of the bleaching agents on mineral loss of enamel

The physical and chemically soundness of the enamel depends on the pH and the saliva consisting of calcium phosphate and fluoride. Caries lesions develop with the fermentation of carbohydrates by bacteria's, the formation of organic acids and the pH decrease. The critical pH value for the enamel is pH= 5.5 and when the oral pH decreases below this value, the bands between the fibrils and apatite of the enamel dissolve and the inorganic structure is affected (Axellson, 2000). In a study (Mcgucking et al., 1992) the enamel surface of bleached teeth were examined with a scanning electron microscope and a profilometer. The results showed that the enamel surface was affected by different concentrated bleaching agents, but these differences were not related with the pH values of the agents. When Tezel *et al* (Tezel et al., 2011; Tezel et al., 2007) measured the pH values of the bleaching agents used in their study with a pH meter it had been found that the pH was approximately 8 for each group. The pH values of bleaching materials were almost similar in the study, but the Ca^{2+} losses of the groups were found to be different. For this reason, they postulated that the pH values of the bleaching agents might not be effective on the Ca^{2+} loss of the groups and that the results were compatible with the study mentioned above.

4. Effects of topical fluoride agents on enamel surface in cooperation with bleaching agents

Considering enamel abrasion, the calcium/phosphate precipitation from saliva results in hardening of porous enamel which gradually may return to its initial situation if the process continues. The amount of the fluoride in the tooth's surface is also an important factor for the changes that could occur after the bleaching process. It has been shown that fluoride has the potential to inhibit demineralization which means that less surface changes would occur. To avoid these unfavorable effects of bleaching treatments, it is recommended to use fluoride containing remineralization agent incorporation with bleaching agents in order to decrease surface solubility (Akal N et al., 2001; Chen et al.,2008)

Taking this suggestion into consideration Tezel *et al* (Tezel et al., 2011) used artificial saliva to reflect the oral conditions and "after bleaching mousse" containing fluoride to maintain clinical schedule in their study mentioned above. This procedure gave them the potential effects of the topical fluoride agent for remineralization. As mentioned before, fluoride has been admitted to remineralize softened enamel by increasing resistance to acid attacks by forming a calcium fluoride layer to inhibit demineralization (Attin et al., 1997; Ten Cate&Arends,1977; Featherstone et al.,1982). It accumulates in the plaque fluid and as calcium fluoride on the enamel surface. During the acid challenge, calcium fluoride is dissolved (Axellson, 2000). It may be a question if the calcium loss could be from the dissolved calcium fluoride or not. Fundamentally, the source of calcium for calcium fluoride is from the enamel. Depending on this fact, the measured calcium loss after the acidic challenge should be from the enamel either directly or indirectly from the dissolved calcium flouride. Nevertheless, further studies are required to estimate this fact.

In another study (Tezel et al., edited to be published) which is still being edited to be published, the effects of different fluoride agents on the caries-like lesion formation and Ca^{2+} loss from the enamel surfaces after bleaching with 38% hydrogen peroxide have been examined. Teeth were divided into four pieces and randomly divided into four groups; three of them being the test groups and the last one being the control. The test groups were then bleached with 38% hydrogen peroxide leaving the control group untreated. Then two out of three test groups were treated with fluoride agents with different concentrations; 1% titanium tetrafluoride (TiF_4) and 1.1% sodium flouride (NaF). Immediately after the application of the bleaching and fluoride agents for prescribed time, the specimens of each group were subjected to erosive demineralization with acetic acid buffered with 0.34M sodium acetate (pH=4). The specimens were demineralized four times for four days. The amount of Ca^{2+} released from the specimens was detected with atomic absorption spectrometer. When the results were examined it was clearly observed that there was a decrease in the Ca^{2+} release in the fluoride-treated groups after bleaching. When these two groups (TiF_4 and NaF) were compared, it was determined that at the end of the test period (16 days) the amount of Ca^{2+} in the buffer solution of TiF_4-treated samples was less than that of NaF-treated samples and the difference was statistically significant (Table 5, 6). Regarding this result, it can be assumed that TiF_4 may be effective in preventing the bleached enamel surface against the acid attacks. Furthermore, there was no Ca^{2+} release from three specimens during the first four days, and during the second 4-day interval. This result can be a result of the glaze layer formed just after the application of TiF_4.

	N		4th Day	8th Day	12th Day	16th Day	Total
Control Group	10	Mean	3.59	3.20	3.72	4.55	15.07
		Std Dev	0.54	0.59	1.23	0.89	1.81
		Min.	3.01	2.46	2.46	2.74	12.60
		Max.	4.93	4.38	6.58	5.75	18.36
38% HP	10	Mean	5.75	5.18	5.56	5.95	22.44
		Std Dev	1.60	1.52	0.71	0.37	2.52
		Min.	3.83	3.01	4.66	5.48	18.36
		Max.	7.95	8.50	6.85	6.58	27.68
38% HP+ NaF	10	Mean	2.05	3.15	3.94	4.52	13.67
		Std Dev	0.83	0.58	1.01	0.83	1.86
		Min.	0.82	2.19	2.46	3.29	10.68
		Max.	3.01	4.11	5.75	6.03	15.61
38% HP+ TiF$_4$	10	Mean	1.15	1.94	2.66	3.37	9.12
		Std Dev	0.92	1.54	0.63	0.48	2.40
		Min.	0	0	1.64	2.46	4.93
		Max.	2.46	4.11	3.56	3.83	11.50

Table 5. Ca^{2+} release from the bleached specimens treated with 1% TiF_4 and 1.1% NaF in mm^2 ($\mu g/ml$).

In a previous study, Tezel *et al* (Tezel et al., 2002) reported that TiF_4 was found to be more effective than Duraphat (NaF, 2.26% F) or Elmex (amine fluoride, 1.25% F) in preventing artificial enamel lesion formation. Attin *et al* (Attin et al., 1999) reported that, fluoridation was effective in increasing resistance of enamel against demineralization by erosive substances. Similarly, the findings of this present study demonstrated that the resistance of enamel against the erosive demineralization caused by 38% HP application was increased after 1% TiF_4 treatment.

When the Ca^{2+} losses from the test groups which were bleached with 38% HP were compared, there was also a decrease in Ca^{2+} losses of 1.1% NaF treated group indicating that NaF could also prevent enamel surfaces against acid attacks during the first four days (p<0.05). Addition of sodium fluoride to hydrogen peroxide solutions leads to formation of fluoridated hydroxyapatite and calcium fluoride when applied on hydroxyapatite samples (Tanizawa, 2005). In the present study, although NaF was effective against acid attacks on enamel surfaces, its influence was not as strong as TiF_4 (Table 6; Figure 8).

Materials	4th Day	8thDay	12th Day	16th Day	Total
Control X 38% HP	*	*	*	*	*
Control X 38% HP + NaF	*	NS	NS	NS	NS
Control X 38% HP + TiF₄	*	NS	NS	*	*
38% HP X 38% HP + NaF	*	*	*	*	*
38% HP 38 X 38 % HP + TiF₄	*	*	*	*	*
38% HP + NaF X 38% HP + TiF₄	NS	NS	*	*	*
* Statistically significant differences between the groups (p<.05) NS No statistically significant differences (p>.05)					

Table 6. Statistical differences between test groups.

Different topical fluoride agents (sodium fluoride, acidulated phosphate fluoride, stannous fluoride, amine fluoride or titanium tetrafluoride) to human tooth enamel are widely used in caries prevention. Topically applied fluoride may reduce the solubility of the surface enamel, render the tooth surface harder, more resistant to demineralization, and more prone to remineralization (Skartveit et al., 1990). The inhibiting effect of sodium fluoride on caries is well documented and a protective effect against dental erosion has been shown *in vitro* (Sorvari et al., 1994; Ganss et al., 2001). Fluoride varnishes provide long contact periods between the dental tissues and the fluoride agent resulting in high fluoride uptake and the formation of calcium fluoride deposits that act as fluoride reservoirs (Arends J & Schuthof, 1975; Grobler et al.,1983; de Bruyn,1987; Petersson,1993). It has been reported that during the application of titanium tetrafluoride, a glaze layer was formed on the tooth surface (Mundorff et al., 1972). TiF_4, has been shown to reduce articifial caries lesion formation and enamel solubility enabling high fluoride uptake (Tezel et al.,2002; Büyükyılmaz et al., 1997).

Generally, fluoride uptake in demineralised enamel is higher when compared to sound enamel (Attin et al., 2006) It is assumed that the porous structure of the demineralised enamel allows better diffusion and penetration of the applied fluoride and that the porosity offers a higher number of possible retention sites for the fluoride. The application of highly concentrated fluoride favors the formation of the calcium-fluoride like layer (Attin et al., 1977). This deposit is later dissolved, allowing fluoride diffuse into the underlying enamel, the saliva, or a plaque layer covering the tooth. It is assumed that some of the fluoride is supporting the remineralization of the enamel. The results of a previous study confirmed that the calcium fluoride layer on the enamel was coated by phosphates and proteins from saliva as a pH-controlling reservoir that acts to decrease demineralization and promote remineralization (Rolla&Saxegaard, 1990).

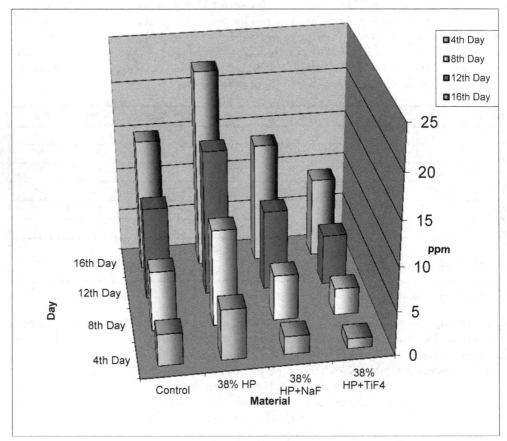

Fig. 8. Cumulative calcium (Ca^{2+}) release from the bleached specimens in the buffer solution after treatment with 1% TiF_4 and 1.1% NaF on the 4th, 8 th, 12 th and 16 th days (µg/ml).

VanRijkom et al (VanRijkom et al., 2003) compared the erosion-inhibiting effect of the topical fluoride treatment based on the deposition of CaF_2-like material using 1% NaF and 4% TiF_4. It was concluded that the reduction of Ca^{2+} loss was more stable for TiF_4 than the NaF group and the reduction appeared to be smaller for the longer acid exposure times. Recently, Magalhães et al (Magalhães et al., 2008) have stated that a TiF_4 varnish showed better results than 2 commercial NaF varnishes in reducing enamel erosion. Based on the results of Tezel *et al*'s (Tezel et al., edited to be published) study, it was shown that topical fluoride applications decreased Ca^{2+} loss from the 38% HP treated enamel surfaces. It may be concluded that the application of fluoride agents may reduce the risk of erosion-like lesions caused by bleaching and remineralize the bleached enamel surfaces. The findings of this in vitro study demonstrated that TiF_4 may act better than NaF solution in preventing acid attacks.

5. Conclusion

As a conclusion, considering the conditions tested, the changes in enamel were directly proportional to the treatment time and peroxide concentration. According to the methodologies used in these studies, higher concentrations of HP caused more Ca^{2+} loss than lower concentrations. The contact time of high concentrated bleaching agents may also be an important factor for Ca^{2+} loss. A recommendation to use activation methods which shorten the contact time of the highly concentrated bleaching agents can be used in the dental office. But it must still be mentioned that 10% CP would be the safest method. In addition, to avoid the unfavorable effects of bleaching treatments, it is recommended to use topical fluoride agents incorporation with bleaching agents to take advantage of remineralization process.

The findings of these *in vitro* studies may not be representative of the *in vivo* condition; in which the oral cavity is continually bathed with saliva that contains various minerals (*i.e.* fluoride, calcium phosphate), lipids, carbohydrates and proteins. They also do not represent unfavorable conditions where the deficiency of saliva or poor oral hygiene that might increase the caries risks. Further studies are needed to clarify the effects of these materials on Ca^{2+} loss of enamel and caries susceptibility.

6. References

Akal, N., Over, H., Olmez, A., & Bodur, H. (2001). Effects of carbamide peroxide containing bleaching agents on the morphology and subsurface hardness of enamel. *J Clin Pediatr Dent,* 25, 4, 293-296.

Arends, J., & Schuthof, J. (1975). Fluoride content in human enamel after fluoride application and washing-an in vitro study. *Caries Res,* 9, 363-372.

Attin, T., Kielbassa, AM., Schawanenberg, M., & Hellwig E. (1997). The effect of fluoride treatment on remineralization of bleached enamel. *J Oral Rehabil,* 24, 282-286.

Attin, T., Deifuss, H., & Hellwig, E. (1999). Influence of acidified fluoride gel on abrasion resistance of eroded enamel. *Caries Res,* 33, 135-139.

Attin, T., Albrecht, K., Becker, K., Hannig, C., & Wiegand, A. (2006). Influence of carbamide peroxide on enamel fluoride uptake. *J Dent,* 34, 668-675.

Axellson, P. (2000). Development and diagnosis of carious lesions. *Diagnosis and Risc Prediction of Dental Caries,* Quintessence, Germany.

Axellson, P. (2000). International Modifiying Factors Involved in Dental Caries (Chapter 3). *In:Diagnosis and Risc Prediction of Dental Caries.* Quintessence Publishing Co, Germany

Basting, RT., Rodrigues, AL Jr., & Serra, MC. (2001). The effect of 10% carbamide peroxide bleaching material on microhardness of sound and demineralized enamel and dentin in situ. *Oper Dent*, 26, 531-539.

Bitter, NC. (1992). A scanning electron microscopy study of the effect of bleaching agents on enamel: A preliminary report. *J Prosthet Dent*, 67, 852-855.

Bitter, NC., & Sanders, JL. (1993). The effect of four bleaching agents on the enamel surface: a scanning electron microscopic study. *Quintessence Int*, 24, 817-824.

Büyükyılmaz, T., Øgaard, B., Duschner, H., Ruben J., & Arends, J. (1997). The caries-preventive effect of titanium tetrafluoride on root surfaces in situ as evaluated by microradiography and confocal laser scanning microscopy. *Adv Dent Res*, 11, 448-452.

Chen, HP., Chang, CH., Chuang, SF., & Yang, JY. (2008). Effect of fluoride containing bleaching agents on enamel surface properties. *J Dent*, 36, 718-725.

Chen, JH., Xu, JW., & Shing, CX. (1993). Decomposition rate of hydrogen peroxide bleaching agents under various chemical and physical conditions. *J Prosthet Dent*, 69,1,46-48.

Davidson, CL., Boom, G., & Arends, J. (1973). Calcium distribution in human and bovine surface enamel. *Caries Res*, 7, 349-359.

de Bruyn, H. (1987). Fluoride Varnishes and Enamel Caries, *PhD thesis*, Groningen.

Featherstone, JD., Cutress, TW., Rodgers, BE., & Dennison, PJ. (1982). Remineralization of artificial caries-like lesions *in vivo* by a self-administered mouthrinse or paste. *Caries Research*, 16(3), 235-42.

Flaitz, CM., & Hicks, MJ. (1996). Effects of carbamide peroxide whitening agents on enamel surface and caries like lesion formation: A SEM and polarized light microscopic *in vitro* study. *J Dent Child*, 63, 249-256.

Ganss, C., Klimek, J., Schaffer, U., & Spall, T. (2001). Effectiveness of two fluoridation measures on erosion progress in human enamel and dentine in vitro. *Caries Res*, 35, 325-330.

Goldstein, GR., & Garber, DA. (1995). Complete Dental Bleaching. Chiacago: *Quintessence Int*.

Grobler, SR., Øgaard, B., & Rølla, G. (1983). Fluoride uptake and retention by sound enamel after in vivo Duraphat application. *J Dent Assoc S Afr*, 38, 55-58.

Haywood, VB. (1992). History, safety and effectiveness of current bleaching techniques and applications of the nightguard vital bleaching technique. *Quintessence Int*, 23, 471-488.

Haywood, VB., & Heymann, HO. (1989). Nightguard vital bleaching. *Quintessence Int*, 20, 173-176.

Haywood, VB., Leech, T., Heymann, HO., Crumpler, D., & Bruggers, K. (1990). Nightguard vital bleaching: effects on enamel surface texture and diffusion. *Quintessence Int*, 21, 801-804.

Hegedüs, C., Bistey, T., Flora-Nagy, E., Keszthelyi, G., & Jenei, A. (1999). An atomic force microscopy study on the effect of bleaching agents on enamel surface. *J Dent*, 27, 509-515.

Hosaya, N., Honda, K., Iino, F., & Arai, T. (2003). Changes in enamel surface roughness and adhesion of *Streptococcus mutans* to enamel after vital bleaching. *J Dent*, 31, 543-548.

Imfeld, T. (1996). Dental erosion. Definition, classification and links. *Eur J Oral Sci,* 104, 151-155.

Ingram, GS., & Fejerskov, O. (1986). A scanning electron microscope study of artificial caries lesion formation. *Caries Res,* 20, 32-39.

Justino, LM., Tames, DR., & Demarco, FF. (2004). In situ and *in vitro* effects of bleaching with carbamide peroxide on human enamel. *Oper Dent,* 29, 2, 219-25.

Lewinstein, I., Hirschfeld, Z., Stabholz, A., & Rotstein, I. (1994). Effect of hydrogen peroxide and sodium perboride on the microhardness of human enamel and dentin. *J Endod,* 20, 61-63.

Lopes, GC., Bonissoni, L., Baratieri, LN., Vieira, LC., & Monteiro, S. (2002). Effect of bleaching agents on the hardness and morphology of enamel. *J Esthet Restor Dent,* 14, 1, 24-30.

Magalhães, AC., Kato, MT., Rios, D., Wiegand, A., Attin, T., & Buzalaf, MAR. (2008). The Effect of an Experimental 4% TiF$_4$ varnish compared to NAF varnishes and 4% TiF$_4$ solution on dental erosion in vitro. *Caries Res,* 42, 269-274.

McGuckin, RS., Babin, JF., & Meyer, BJ. (1992). Alteration in human enamel surface morphology following vital bleaching. *J Prosthet Dent,* 68(5), 754-60.

Mundorff, SA., Little, MF., & Bibby, BG. (1972). Enamel dissolution: II. Action of titanium tetrafluoride. *J Dent Res,* 51, 1567-1571.

Murchinson, DF., Charlton, DG., & Moore, BK. (1992). Carbamide peroxide bleaching: Effects on enamel surface hardness and bonding. *Oper Dent,* 17, 181-185.

Perdigão, J., Francci, C., Swift Jr EJ., Ambrosse WW., & Lopes M. (1998). Ultra-morphological study of the interaction of dental adhesives with carbamide peroxide-bleached enamel. *Am J Dent,* 11, 291-301.

Petersso, LG. (1993). Fluoride mouthrinses and fluoride varnishes. *Caries Res,* 27,(suppl 1), 35-42.

Potocnick, I., Kosec ,L., & Gaspersic, D. (2000), Effect of 10% carbamide peroxide bleaching gel on enamel microhardness, microstructure and mineral content. *J Endod,* 26, 203-206.

Quirynen, M., & Bollen, CM. (1995). The influence of surface roughness and surface free-energy on supra-and sub-gingival plaque formation in man. A review of the literature. *J Clin Periodontol,* 22, 1–14.

Rodrigues, JA., Basting, RT., Serra, MC., & Rodrigues, AL Jr. (2001). Effects of 10% carbamide peroxide bleaching materials on enamel microhardness. *Am J Dent,* 14, 67-71.

Rølla, G., & Saxegaard, E. (1990). Critical evaluation of the composition and use of topical fluorides with the emphasis on the role of calcium fluoride in caries inhibition. *J Dent Res,* 69, 780-785.

Rotstein, I., Danker, E., Goldman, A., Helling, I., Stahbolz, A., & Zalkind, M. (1996). Histochemical analysis of dental hard tissues following bleaching. *J Endod,* 22, 23-25.

Seghi RR., & Denhy, I. (1992). Effects of external bleaching on indentation and abrasion characteristics of human enamel in vitro. *J Dent Res,* 71, 1340-1344.

Skartveit, L., Knut, AS., Myklebust, S., &Tveit, AB. (1990). Effect of TiF$_4$ solutions on bacterial growth in vitro and on tooth surfaces. *Acta Odontol Scand*, 48, 169-174.

Smidt, A., Weller, D., Roman, I., & Gedalia, J. (1998). Effect of bleaching agents on microhardness and surface morphology of tooth enamel. *Am J Dent*, 11, 83-85.

Sorvari, R., Meurman, JH., Alakuijala, P., & Frank, RM. (1994). Effect of fluoride varnish and solution on enamel in vitro. *Caries Res*, 28, 227-32.

Spalding, M., Taveira, LA., & de Assis, GF. (2003). Scanning electron microscopy study of dental enamel surface exposed to 35% hydrogen peroxide: alone, with saliva, and with 10% carbamide peroxide. *J Esthet Restor Dent*, 15, 3, 154-64.

Sydney, GB., Barletta, FB., & Sydney, RB. (2002). *In vitro* analysis of effects of heat used in dental bleaching on human dental enamel. *Braz Dent J*, 13, 166-169.

Tanizawa, Y. (2005). Reaction characteristics of a tooth-bleaching agent containing H$_2$O$_2$ and NaF: in vitro study of crystal structure change in treated hydoxyapatite and chemical states of incorporated fluorine. *Int J Cosm Sci*, 56, 121-134.

Ten Cate, JM., & Arends, J. (1977). Remineralization of artificial enamel lesions in vitro. *Caries Research*, 11(5), 277-86

Tezel, H., Atalayin, C., Erturk, O., & Karasulu, E. (2011). Susceptibility of enamel treated with bleaching agents to mineral loss after cariogenic challenge. *International Journal of Dentistry*, 2011, Article ID 953835, 8 pages doi:10.1155/2011/953835

Tezel, H., Ergücü, Z., & Önal, B. (2002). Effects of topical fluoride agents on artificial enamel lesion formation in vitro. *Quintessence Int*, 33, 347-352.

Tezel, H., Ergücü, Z., & Söğüt, Ö. (editted to be published). The effects of titanium tetrafluoride and sodium fluoride on calcium loss from bleached enamel.

Tezel, H., Ertaş, SÖ., Özata, F., Dalgar, H., & Korkut, Z. (2007). Effect of bleaching agent on calcium loss from the enamel surface. *Quintessence Int*, 38, 4, 339-347.

Titley, K., Torneck, CD., & Smith, DC. (1998). The effect of concentrated hydrogen peroxide solutions on the surface morphology of human tooth enamel. *J Endodont*, 14, 69-74.

Türkun, M., Sevgican, F., Pehlivan, Y., & Aktener, BO. (2002). Effects of 10% carbamide peroxide on the enamel surface morphology: a scanning electron microscopy study. *J Esthet Restor Dent*, 14, 4, 238-44.

Van Rijkom, H., Ruben, J., Vieira, A., Huysmans, MC., Truin, GJ., & Mulder, J. (2003). Erosion-inhibiting effect of sodium fluoride and titanium tetrafluoride treatment in vitro. *Eur J Oral Sci*, 111, 253-257.

Wetter, NU., Barroso, MCS., & Pelino, JEP. (2004). Dental bleaching efficacy with diode laser and LED irradiation: an *in vitro* study. *Lasers Surg Med*, 35, 254-258.

Zalkind, M., Arwaz, JR., Goldman, A., & Rotstein, I. (1996). Surface morphology changes in human enamel, dentin and cementum following bleaching: A scanning electron microscopy study. *Endod Dent Traumatol*, 12, 82-88.

Zhang, C., Wang, X., Kinoshita, JI., Zhao, B., Toko, T., & Kimura, Y. (2007). Effect of KTP laser irradiation, diode laser, and LED on tooth bleaching: a comparative study. *Photomed Laser Surg*, 25, 91-95.

5

Statistical Models for Dental Caries Data

David Todem

Division of Biostatistics, Department of Epidemiology and Biostatistics,
Michigan State University, East Lansing, MI,
USA

1. Introduction

Tooth decay is ubiquitous among humans and is one of the most prevalent oral diseases. Although this condition is largely preventable, more than half of all adults over the age of eighteen present early signs of the disease, and at some point in life about three out of four adults will develop the disease. Tooth decay is also common among children as young as five and remains the most common chronic disease of children aged five to seventeen years. It is estimated that tooth decay is four times more prevalent than asthma in childhood (Todem, 2008). Tooth decay and its correlates such as poor oral health place an enormous burden on the society. Poor oral health and a propensity to dental caries have been related to decreased school performance, poor social relationships and less success later in life. It is estimated that about 51 million school hours per year are lost in the U.S. alone because of dental-related illness. In older adults, tooth decay is one of the leading causes of tooth loss which has a dramatic impact on chewing ability leading to detrimental changes in food selection. This, in turn, may increase the risk of systemic diseases such as cardiovascular diseases and cancer.

The etiology of dental caries is well established. It is a localized, progressive demineralization of the hard tissues of the crown and root surfaces of teeth. The demineralization is caused by acids produced by bacteria, particularly mutans Streptococci and possibly Lactobacilli, that ferment dietary carbohydrates. This occurs within a bacteria-laden gelatinous material called dental plaque that adheres to tooth surfaces and becomes colonized by bacteria. Thus, dental caries results from the interplay of three main factors over time: dietary carbohydrates, cariogenic bacteria within dental plaque, and susceptible hard tooth surfaces. Dental caries is also a dynamic process since periods of demineralization alternate with periods of remineralization through the action of fluoride, calcium and phosphorous contained in oral fluids.

The evaluation of the severity of tooth decay is often performed at the tooth surface level. According to the World Health Organization, both the shape and the depth of a carious lesion at the tooth surface level can be scored on a four-point scale, D_1 to D_4. Level D_1 refers to clinically detectable enamel lesions with non-cavitated surfaces; D_2 for clinically detectable cavities limited to the enamel; D_3 for clinically detectable lesions in dentin; and finally D_4 for lesions into the pulp. Despite these detailed tooth-level data, most epidemiological studies often rely on the decayed, missing and filled (DMF) index, developed in the 1930s by Klein *et al.* (see for example Klein and Palmer, 1938). This index is applied to all the teeth (DMFT) or to all surfaces (DMFS), and represents the cumulative severity of dental caries experience for each individual. These scores have well documented shortcomings regarding their ability to describe the intra-oral distribution of dental caries (Lewsey and Thomson, 2004). But they continue to be instrumental in evaluating and comparing the risks of dental caries across population groups. Most importantly, they remain popular in dental caries research for their ability to conduct historical comparisons in population-based studies.

Statistical analysis of dental caries data relies heavily on the research question under study. These questions can be classified into two groups. The first group represents questions that can be answered using mouth-level outcomes generated using aggregated scores such as the DMF index. The second group refers to questions that necessitate the use of tooth or tooth-surface level outcomes. A very important issue to address for the data analyst is the modeling strategy to adopt for the response variable under investigation. Broadly, two fairly different views are advocated. The first view, supported by large-sample properties, states that normal theory should be applied as much as possible, even to non-normal data such as counts (Verbeke and Molenberghs, 2000). This view is strengthened by the notion that, normal models, despite being a member of the generalized linear models (GLIM), are much further developed than any other GLIM (e.g. model checks and diagnostic tools), and that they enjoy unique properties (e.g., the existence of closed form solutions, exact distributions for test statistics, unbiased estimators, etc...). Although this is correct in principle, it fails to acknowledge that normal models may not be adequate for some types of data. As an example, the abundance of zeros in DMF scores rules out any attempt to use normal models, such as linear models, even after a suitable transformation. While a transformation may normalize the distribution of nonzero response values, no transformation could spread the zeros (Hall, 2000). A different modeling view is that each type of outcome should be analyzed using tools that exploit the nature of the data. For dental data, features to be accommodated include the discrete nature of the data (count responses for mouth-level data and binary response for intra-oral data), the abundance of zeros for example in the DMF/S scoring, and the clustering in intra-oral responses. The clustering of participants as a result of the study design is another important feature.

This chapter reviews common statistical parametric models to answer questions that arise in dental caries research, with an eye to discerning their relative strengths and limitations. Missing data problems arising in caries dental reasrch will also be discussed but touched on briefly.

2. Statistical models for mouth-level caries data

Mouth-level data, resulting from the DMF index, are typically analyzed as unbounded or bounded counts. For unbounded counts, a Poisson regression model or its extension the negative binomial regression model that accounts for overdispersion in the data, are often used. A binomial regression model for bounded counts is often advocated.

For unbounded counts, these models assume that the basic underlying distribution for the data is either a Poisson or a negative binomial distribution. The Poisson model is the simplest distribution for nonnegative discrete data, and is entirely specified by a positive parameter the mean. This mean is often related to potential explanatory variables using a log link function. Specifically, let Y define the outcome variable and X the set of explanatory variables. A Poisson regression model for the mean is defined as $E(Y|X) = e^{\alpha+X\beta}$, where α and β are the intercept and the regression parameter vector associated with X. The probability mass function of Y is given by: $P(Y = y|X) = \frac{e^{-\mu_x}\mu_x^y}{\Gamma(y+1)}$, y=0,1,..., where $\mu_x = E(Y|X)$ is the conditional mean which depends on covariates.

One major restriction of the Poisson regression model is that its mean is equal to its variance. For dental caries data, however, it is not uncommon for the variance to be much greater than the mean. For such data, a negative binomial regression model has been advocated as an alternative to Poisson regression models. It is typically used when the variability in the data cannot be properly captured by Poisson regression models. The negative binomial model is a conjugate mixture distribution for count data (Agresti, 2002). It is entirely specified by two parameters, its mean and the overdispersion parameter. Similarly to the Poisson regression model, the mean is related to potential explanatory variables using a log link function. However, the probability mass function of Y is given by:

$$P(Y = y|X) = \frac{\Gamma(y + \kappa^{-1})}{\Gamma(\kappa^{-1})\Gamma(y + 1)} \left(\frac{\kappa^{-1}}{\mu_x + \kappa^{-1}}\right)^{\kappa^{-1}} \left(1 - \frac{\kappa^{-1}}{\mu_x + \kappa^{-1}}\right)^y, \qquad y = 0,1,...$$

where $\mu_x = E(Y|X) = e^{\alpha+X\beta}$ is the conditional mean which depends on covariates, and κ is the overdispersion parameter. This distribution has variance $\mu_x + \kappa\mu_x^2$. Parameter κ is typically unknown and estimated from data to evaluate the extent of overdispersion in the data. When κ tends to zero, the negative binomial model converges to a Poisson process (Agresti, 2002).

The presence of an upper bound for possible values taken by DMF scores suggests a model based on the binomial rather than the Poisson distribution (Hall, 2000). Data are then viewed as being generated from a binomial process with m trials and success probability π_X. Here m represents the maximum number of teeth or tooth surfaces in the mouth susceptible to decay, and π_X the probability for a tooth or tooth surface to present a sign of decay. The binomial model is given by:

$$P(Y = y|X) = \frac{\Gamma(m + 1)}{\Gamma(m - y + 1)\Gamma(y + 1)} (\pi_X)^y (1 - \pi_X)^{m-y}, y = 0,1, ... m,$$

where the success probability is related to covariates as $\pi_X = \frac{e^{\alpha+X\beta}}{1+e^{\alpha+X\beta}}$, with α and β being the intercept and the regression parameter vector associated with X. One should note however that Poisson and negative binomial distributions provide a reasonable approximation to the binomial distribution in dental caries research.

Dental caries data with excess zeros are common in statistical practice. For example, in young children, DMF scores generally generate an excessive number of zeros in that many children do not experience dental caries. This is typically due to a short exposure time to caries development. The limitations of Poisson and negative binomial regression models to analyze such data are well established (see, for example, Lambert, 1992; and Hall, 2000). One approach to analyze count data with many zeros is to use zero-inflated models. This class of models views the data as being generated from $P(Y = y|X)$ a mixture of a zero point mass and a non-degenerate homogenous discrete distribution $P_1(Y = y|X)$ as follows:

$$P(Y = y|X) = \begin{cases} \omega + (1 - \omega)P_1(Y = y|X), & y = 0 \\ (1 - \omega)P_1(Y = y|X), & y > 0, \end{cases}$$

where $0 \leq \omega \leq 1$ represents the mixing probability that captures the heterogeneity of zeros in the population. The choice of the homogenous distribution $P_1(Y = y|X)$ for the most part depends on the nature of counts under consideration. For bounded counts, a binomial distribution is typically used (Hall, 2000). Poisson and negative binomial distributions are the standard for unbounded counts (Bohning et al., 1999). Ridout, Demetrio and Hinde (1998) provide an extensive review of this literature. In real applications of these models in dental caries research, the mixing probability is often related to covariates using for example a logistic model.

We illustrate below how some of these simple models can be applied to dental caries scores data generated from a survey designed to collect oral health information on low-income African American children (0-5 years), living in the city of Detroit (see Tellez et al., 2006). This study aimed at promoting oral health and reducing its disparities within this community through the understanding of determinants of dental caries. Dental caries were measured using DMF scores which represent the cumulative severity of the disease for each surveyed participants. Possible covariates include the study participant's age (AGE) and his/her sugar intake (SI). In Table 1, we present the fitted regression models applied to children's data. For these data, the mean structure of the homogeneous model is specified as $E(Y|X) = e^{\alpha + X\beta}$, where $X = (AGE, SI, AGE * SI)$, with $AGE * SI$ being a multiplicative interaction, and $\beta = (\beta_1, \beta_2, \beta_3)'$. Parameter κ of the Negative Binomial model captures overdispersion in data.

Parameter	Homogeneous Poisson	Homogeneous Negative Binomial	Zero-inflated Negative Binomial (mixing weight depends on covariates)
α	1.3994(0.0209)*	1.3484(0.0725)*	2.0158(0.0676)*
β_1	0.6981(0.0193)*	0.9188(0.0861)*	0.2350(0.0679)*
β_2	0.2696(0.0203)*	0.2378(0.0853)*	0.0573(0.0695)
β_3	-0.2790(0.0219)*	-0.3314(0.0877)*	-0.0728(0.0739)
γ_0	-	-	-0.6131(0.1595)*
γ_1	-	-	-1.7191(0.2276)*
γ_2	-	-	-0.2226(0.1509)
γ_3	-	-	0.3163(0.2022)
κ	-	2.6178(0.1753)*	0.9295(0.1058)*
-2logLik	8455.7	4059.1	3815.4
AIC	8463.7	4069.1	3833.4

*: p-value<0.05

Table 1. Parameter estimates and (Standard errors) from a homogeneous Poisson model, a homogeneous Negative Binomial model, and a zero-inflated Negative Binomial model with covariate dependent mixing weights applied to DMF scores

As a basic starting model, a homogeneous Poisson regression model is fit and compared to a homogeneous Negative Binomial model. In view of the AIC, the homogeneous Negative Binomial model provides a reasonably good fit compared to the Poisson model. This result is consistent with overdispersion parameter κ in the homogeneous Negative Binomial model being statistically significant at 5%, suggesting that overdispersion cannot be ignored in these data. As a result, the standard errors of parameter estimates in the mean model under the homogeneous Negative Binomial model are larger compared to those of the homogeneous Poisson model. The homogeneous Negative Binomial model is further compared to a zero-inflated Negative Binomial model which potentially accommodates extra zeros in the data. In the latter model, the mixing weight ω is related to covariates as, $\omega = \{1 + e^{-\gamma Z}\}^{-1}$, where $Z = (AGE, SI, AGE * SI)$ and $\gamma = (\gamma_0, \gamma_1, \gamma_2, \gamma_3)'$. In view of the AIC, this model provides a better representation of the data compared to the homogeneous Negative Binomial model. This is consistent with findings from the literature dental caries in young children typically exhibit overdispersion in addition to zero-inflation (Bohning et al, 1999).

The zero-inflated regression models provide an interesting parametric framework to accommodate heterogeneity in a population. A prevailing concern, however, is that these models only accommodate an inflation of zeros in the population. Inflation and deflation at zero often arise in various practical applications. Homogeneous models (Poisson and negative binomial regression models) when applied to data from the Detroit study typically reveal an inflation of zeros (few children with no dental caries predicted than observed) for younger children and deflation of zeros (more children with no dental caries predicted than observed) for older children. For such data, a model that captures only inflation of zeros may fail to properly represent heterogeneity in the population. This then necessitates the use of models that can accommodate both inflation and deflation in the population. A good example of such models is the two-stage model also known as the Hurdle model (Mullahy, 1986). An alternative approach is to use the marginal distribution derived from the mixture distribution:

$$P(Y = y|X) = \begin{cases} \omega + (1 - \omega)P_1(Y = y|X), & y = 0 \\ (1 - \omega)P_1(Y = y|X), & y > 0, \end{cases}$$

where $\frac{-P_1(Y=0|X)}{1-P_1(Y=0|X)} \leq \omega \leq 1$. Note here that the constraints on the mixing weights are obtained only by imposing that, $0 \leq P(Y = y|X) \leq 1$ for all y. The mixing weight is potential negative to accommodate deflation in the data. For this class of models, the marginal mixture model maintains his hierarchical representation only if the mixing weight are bounded between 0 and 1. When the mixing weight is negative, the marginal mixture model then loses its hierarchical representation.

Finally, the models described above are basic starting models and should be extended to accommodate unique features of the data under consideration. For example, it is often the case that the sampling design used to recruit study participants leads to clustered data. In survey research, sampled subjects living in the same neighborhood are more likely to share common, typically unmeasured, predispositions or characteristics that lead to dependent data. This therefore necessitates the use of models for clustered or correlated data. An example of such models is described by Todem et al. (2010) for the analysis of dental caries for low-income African American children under the age of six living in the city of Detroit. These authors extended the family of Poisson and negative binomial models to derive the joint distribution of clustered counted outcomes with extra zeros. Two random effects models were formulated. The first model assumed a shared random effects term between the logistic model of the conditional probability of perfect zeros and the conditional mean of the imperfect state. The second formulation relaxed the shared random effects assumption by relating the conditional probability of perfect zeros and the conditional mean of the imperfect state to two correlated random effects variables. Under the conditional independence assumption and the missing data at random assumption, a direct optimization of the marginal likelihood and an EM algorithm were proposed to fit the proposed models.

3. Statistical models for intra-oral caries data

Although many dental studies provide detailed tooth-level data on caries activity, most analyses still rely on aggregated scores such as the DMF index. These scores summarize at mouth level caries information for each individual typically recorded at the tooth level or tooth-surface level. They have therefore been instrumental in evaluating and comparing the risks for dental caries among population groups. Despite these advances in the etiology of dental caries, there are still some fundamental questions regarding the spatial distribution of dental caries in the mouth that remain unanswered. The intra-oral spatial distribution of dental caries can help answer questions on whether the disease develops symmetrically in the mouth, and whether different types of teeth (Incisors, Canines and Molars) and tooth surfaces (Facial, Lingual, occlusal, Mesial, Distal, and incisal surfaces) are equally susceptible to dental caries. It is well recognized that the different morphology of the pit-and-fissure surfaces of teeth makes them more susceptible to decay than the smooth surfaces. Thus, it is no surprise that the posterior molar and premolar teeth that have pit-and-fissure surfaces are more susceptible to decay than the anterior teeth.

The analysis of intra-oral data poses a number of difficulties due to inherent spatial association of teeth and tooth-surfaces in the mouth. It is well known, for example, that the multiplicity of outcomes recorded on the same unit necessitates the use of methods for correlated data. This section reviews some of the commonly used statistical techniques to analyze such data. A focus will be on parametric models, namely the class of generalized linear mixed effects models and the class of generalized estimating equation models. These regression models take into account the unique spatial structure of teeth and tooth-surfaces in the mouth.

i.   Generalized linear mixed effects models

Generalized linear mixed-effects models constitute the broader class of mixed-effects models for correlated continuous, binary, multinomial and count data (Breslow and Clayton, 1993). They are likelihood-based and often are formulated as hierarchical models. At the first stage, a conditional distribution of the response given random effects is specified, usually assumed to be a member of the exponential family. At the second stage, a prior distribution (typically normal) is imposed on the random effects. The conditional expectations (given random effects) are made of two components, a fixed effects term and a random effects term. The fixed effects term represents covariate effects that do not change with the subject. Random effects represent subject-specific coefficients viewed as deviations from the fixed effects (average) coefficients. Most importantly, they account for the within-mouth correlation under the conditional independence assumption. In dental caries research, data collected at the tooth level or tooth-surface level are typically binary outcomes representing the presence or absence of decay. For such data, a logistic regression model with random effects is typically used. In this class of models, fixed-effects regression parameters have a subject-specific interpretation, conditional on random effects (Verbeke and Molenberghs, 2000). That is, they have a direct and meaningful interpretation only for covariates that change within the cluster level (subject's mouth) such as the location of a tooth or a tooth-surface in the mouth. The probabilities of tooth and tooth-surface decay are conditional given random effects and can be used to capture changes occurring within a particular subject's mouth. To assess changes across all subjects' mouths, the modeler is then required to integrate out the random effects from the quantities of interest. Generalized linear mixed effects models are likelihood-based and therefore can be highly sensitive to any distribution misspecification. But they are known to be robust against less restrictive missing data mechanisms (Little and Rubin, 1987).

ii.   Generalized estimating equations models

Although there are a variety of standard likelihood-based models available to analyze data when the outcome is approximately normal, models for discrete outcomes (such as binary outcomes) generally require a different methodology. Kung-Yee Liang and Scott Zeger (1986) have proposed the so-called Generalized Estimating Equations-GEE model, which is an extension of generalized linear models to correlated data. The basic idea of this family of models is to specify a function that links the linear predictor to the mean response, and use a set of estimating functions with any working correlation model for parameter estimation. A sandwich estimator that corrects for any misspecification of the working correlation model is then used to compute the parameters' standard errors. GEE-based models are very popular as an all-round technique to analyze correlated data when the exact likelihood is difficult to specify. One of the strong points of this methodology is that the full joint distribution of the data does not need to be fully specified to guarantee asymptotically consistent and normal parameter estimates. Instead, a working correlation model between the clustered observations is required for estimation. GEE regression parameter estimates have a population-averaged interpretation, analogous to those obtained from a cross-sectional data analysis. This property makes GEE-based models desirable in population-based studies, where the focus is on average affects accounting for the within-subject association viewed as a nuisance term.

The GEE approach has several advantages over a likelihood-based model. It is computationally tractable in applications where the parametric approaches are computationally very demanding, if not impossible. It is also less sensitive to distribution misspecification as compared to full likelihood-based models. A major limitation of GEE-based models at least in their 1986 original formulation is that they require a more stringent missing data mechanism to produce valid inferences.

4. Conclusion

As the search for effective measures for the prevention and treatment of dental caries continues, it is essential that we have effective, robust and rigorous statistical methods to help our understanding of the condition. This chapter has reviewed common statistical models to answer questions involving intra-oral and mouth-level outcomes, with an eye to discerning their relative strengths and limitations. Models for mouth-level data such as the DMF scores are basically count regression techniques. These models are often extended to two-component distributions when there are excess zeros. This class of models views the data as being generated from a mixture of a zero point mass and a non degenerate discrete distribution. Models for intra-oral outcomes are primarily correlated models for binary data, such as generalized linear mixed effects models and generalized estimating equations models. These models can account for the multilevel data structure (e.g., teeth within a quadrant and quadrants within the mouth) which generate a very complex and unique correlation structure (Zhang et al., 2010). Despite the relative merits of these models to account for the correlation structure, they need to be adapted to accommodate other unique features of intra-oral caries data. Intra-oral data present a unique set of challenges to statistical analysis which includes, but are not limited to, large cluster sizes and informative cluster sizes (Leroux *et al.*, 2006). More generally, models for intra-oral and mouth-level outcomes need to be adapted to the study design. For example, when the study design involves a longitudinal component, the model needs to be adapted accordingly.

Another important issue that needs to be accounted for is that of missing data. This problem is commonly encountered throughout statistical work and is almost ever present in the analysis of dental caries data. Incomplete data can have a dramatic impact on inferences if they are not properly investigated. Using terminology from Little and Rubin (1987), missing data mechanisms are classified as missing completely at random (MCAR), missing at random (MAR) and missing not at random (MNAR), if missingness is allowed to depend (1) none of the outcomes, (2) the observed outcomes only, or (3) unobserved outcomes as well, respectively. GEE-based models at least in their 1986 original formulation require the more stringent MCAR mechanism to produce valid inferences. Weighted GEE-based models have been proposed to accommodate a less stringent missing data mechanism, the missing data at random process (Robins et al., 1995). Likelihood-based models such as generalized linear mixed effects models are known to be robust against the less restrictive MAR mechanism. When the missingness mechanism depends on the unobserved outcomes, these two classes of regression models are likely to produce biased inferences. For example, missing dental caries data generated from missing teeth are likely to be informative in that a missing tooth may be an indication of the severity of the decay for that particular tooth prior to the loss. For such data, ignoring missing data may lead to biased inferences. When a MNAR mechanism is suspected, a model that incorporates both the information from the outcome process and the missing data process into a unified estimating function was advocated (Diggle and Kenward, 1994 and Molenberghs et al. 1997). Such an approach has provoked a large debate about the role for such models in understanding the true data generating mechanism. The original enthusiasm was followed by skepticism about the strong and untestable assumptions on which this type of models rests (Verbeke et al., 2001). Specifically, joint models for the outcomes and missing data are typically not identifiable from observed data at hand. One then has to impose quantitative restrictions to recover identifiability. Conventional restrictions result from considering a minimal set of parameters, called sensitivity parameters, conditional upon which the remaining parameters are assumed identifiable. This method therefore produces a range of models which forms the basis of sensitivity analysis (Vach And Blettner, 1995).

Well established parametric models for dental caries data can be fit with most common statistical software including but not limited to SAS, Splus, R and SPSS. Options are however limited for newly developed models that have emerged in the literature. For recent statistical models in dental caries research to be accepted and used widely, there should be reliable and user-friendly software, readily available to perform regression analysis routinely. The software should be time-efficient, well-documented and most importantly should have a friendly interface, features that are of course closely related to the requirement of being user-friendly. Once these regression models are implemented, this will help answer both mouth-level and questions in population-based research.

Keywords: Generalized estimating equation models, Generalized linear mixed effects models, Negative Binomial models, Poisson models, Zero-inflated models for count data

5. References

Agresti, A. (2002), *Categorical Data Analysis*, Second Edition, New York: John Wiley & Sons.

Breslow, N. E. and Clayton, D. G. Approximate inference in generalized linear mixed models. *J. Amer. Statist. Assoc.*, 88:9–25, 1993.

Bohning, D., Dietz, E., Schlattmann, P., Mendonca, L. and Kirchner, U. (1999). The zero-inflated poisson model and the decayed, missing and filled teeth index in dental epidemiology. *Journal of the Royal Statistical Society: Series A (Statistics in Society)* 162, 195–209.

Diggle, P. & Kenward, M. G. (1994). Informative dropout in longitudinal data analysis (with discussion). *Applied Statistics* 43, 49–93.

Hall, D. B. (2000). Zero-inflated Poisson and binomial regression with random effects: A case study. *Biometrics,* 56, 1030–1039.

Klein H, Palmer C (1938). Studies on dental caries vs. familial resemblance in the caries experience of siblings. *Pub Hlth Rep,* 53:1353-1364.

Lambert, D. (1992). Zero-inflated Poisson regression, with an application to defects in manufacturing. *Technometrics* 34, 1–14.

Leroux, B. (2006). Analysis of correlated dental data: challenges and recent developments. *Statistical Methods for Oral Health Research, JSM 2006.*

Liang, K. Y. & Zeger, S. L. (1986). Longitudinal data analysis using generalized linear models. *Biometrika* 73, 13–22.

Little, R. and Rubin, D. (1987). *Statistical analysis with missing data.* New York: John Wiley and Sons.

Lewsey, J. D. and Thomson, W. M. (2004), The utility of the zero-inflated Poisson and zero-inflated negative binomial models: a case study of cross-sectional and longitudinal DMF data examining the effect of socio-economic status, Community Dentistry and Oral Epidemiology, 32:183–189

Molenberghs, G., Kenward, M. G. & Lesaffre, E. (1997). The analysis of longitudinal ordinal data with non-random dropout. *Biometrika* 84, 33–44.

Mullahy, J. 1986. Specification and testing of some modified count data models. Journal of Econometrics 3: 341–365.

Ridout, M., Hinde, J. and Demetrio, C. G. B. (2001). A score test for testing a zero-inflated Poisson regression model against zero-inflated negative binomial alternatives. *Biometrics* 57, 219–223.

Robins, J., Rotnitzky, A. and Zhao, L.P. (1995). Analysis of semiparametric regression models for repeated outcomes under the presence of missing data. *Journal of the American Statistical Association*, 90,106

Tellez, M., Sohn, W., Burt, B.A., & Ismail A. I. (2006). Assessment of the relationship between neighborhood characteristics and dental caries severity among low-income African-Americans: a multilevel approach., *J Public Health Dent*.66:30-6.

Todem, D. (2008). Oral Health. In Sarah Boslaugh (ed.) Encyclopedia of Epidemiology, Sage Publications (vol 2, pp: 762-764), Los Angeles

Todem, D, Zhang, Y., Ismail, A., and Sohn, W. (2010). Random effects regression models for count data with excess zeros in caries research, Journal of Applied Statistics, 37(10): 1661 - 1679

Vach, W. & Blettner, M. (1995). Logistic regression with incompletely observed categorical covariates – Investigating the sensitivity against violation of the missing at random assumption. *Statistics in Medicine* 14, 1315–1329.

Verbeke, C. and Molenberghs, G. (2000) *Linear mixed models for longitudinal data*. New York: Springer-Verlag.

Verbeke, G., Molenberghs, G., Thijs, H., Lesaffre, E. & Kenward, M. (2001). Sensitivity analysis for nonrandom dropout: A local influence approach. *Biometrics* 57, 7–14.

Zhang, Y., D. Todem, K. Kim and E. Lesaffre (2011). Bayesian Latent Variable Models for Spatially Correlated Tooth-level Binary Data in Caries Research, Statistical Modelling, 11(1):25-47

Part 2

The Diagnosis of Caries

6

How to Diagnose Hidden Caries?
The Role of Laser Fluorescence

Camilo Abalos, Amparo Jiménez-Planas,
Elena Guerrero, Manuela Herrera and Rafael Llamas
University of Seville, School Dentistry,
Spain

1. Introduction

The diagnosis of pits, grooves and fissures is one of the main challenges facing dentists in their professional activity, since the existence of an intact enamel surface may hide deep caries in dentin. Lesions of this kind were described by Weerheijm et al. (1992) as "hidden caries". Over 70 years ago a high incidence of caries was confirmed in grooves and fissures (Hyat, 1923), in coincidence with more recent observations (Bragamian & Garcia-Godoy, 2009). In order to understand and explain this high incidence and the morphological peculiarities involved, it is essential to know the physiopathology of the tooth and of the carious lesion.

Caries is a *"multifactorial disease causing dissolution of the organic component and demineralization of the inorganic component of the hard dental tissues"* (Bonilla, 1998). In the chronology of this process is must be noted that the enamel is a filtering membrane allowing the transit of substances from the exterior to the interior, and vice versa (Llamas et al., 2000). This is because the enamel contains areas with increased water and organic material contents, such as the lamellae or cracks, striae of Retzius, adamantine rod sheath, inter-rod space, and inter-crystalline areas, among others. These zones allow the flow of acids from bacterial plaque, giving rise to disintegration of the organic material and posteriorly conditioning demineralization of the inorganic component – thus supporting the proteolysis – chelation theory of dental caries. These enamel areas with disintegration of the organic material, and the large structural defects such as cracks, which are rich in organic material, can facilitate the penetration of bacteria into deep areas of the enamel, without the existence of superficial cavitation (Brännstrom et al., 1980).

The unpredictable, irregular and varied morphology of the grooves and fissures is well known and makes it impossible to pre-determine the structure; however, it is known that over 50% of all studied teeth have cracks in the depths of the fissures that facilitate the rapid transit of substances and/or bacteria from the depth of the sulcus to the dentin (Pastor et al., 1998). On furthermore considering that enamel thickness from the depth of the sulcus to the dentin is variable and in some cases inexistent, it can be understood why a carious lesion beginning within a fissure can develop in enamel and even in dentin without any external clinical or morphological signs of caries. This in turn explains how in some cases we can observe grooves and fissures that are apparently normal or with a discrete brown or blackish color, but with no cavitations reflecting an incipient or consolidated lesion affecting even the dentin (Fig.1). In view of the above, how can we know if we are dealing with a true initial dentinal carious lesion if the tooth appears to be healthy? Or how can we diagnose something in depth based on the surface appearance? On the other hand, how and when do we decide to open the fissure or not? If we fail to open the fissure dentin caries may exist and progress rapidly; alternatively, a decision to open the fissure may cause us to needlessly damage an intact tooth. We thus face a diagnostic dilemma.

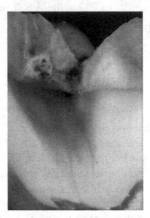

Fig. 1. Non-cavitated occlusal caries with deep dentin involvement.

This problem could be a minor concern if the disorder in question were of low prevalence. However, despite the decrease in the frequency of caries in the industrialized world over the last 20 years (Mejàre et al., 2004), not all clinical forms of caries have evolved equally; indeed, caries of grooves and fissures are those showing the greatest prevalence at the present time, since the most notorious decrease has corresponded to caries of smooth surface (Bagramian & Garcia-Godoy, 2009). The form of presentation has also changed; in effect, enamel presently takes longer in becoming affected, thanks mainly to continuous exposure to fluor. As a result, caries develops more slowly, with preservation of enamel integrity for longer periods of time. At present, caries of grooves and fissures affect between 10-50% of the permanent molars of adolescents (Weerheijm et al., 1992), these being the locations where most carious lesions are found, and non-cavitation persists for a longer period of time. Based on the above, it can be concluded that we are not only facing a diagnostic problem, with a high prevalence in adolescents and young adults, but are also facing a buccodental health problem.

The objective of modern Odontology should be to ensure the prevention of caries, avoiding invasive treatments as far as possible. However, this is only possible if full restitution of the affected tissue is achieved (Hibst et al., 2001). In this context, diagnostic tools should evolve in order to allow us to detect the first signs of enamel demineralization. In other words, the tendency should be to facilitate the early detection of caries, with a view to adopting noninvasive treatments and the corresponding preventive measures. On the other hand, we fundamentally should center on common diagnostic techniques that are accessible to dentists, in order for such strategies to be applicable to routine clinical practice.

2. Diagnostic tests

The existing means for the diagnosis of non-cavitary occlusal caries of grooves and fissures are diverse in terms of the underlying principles and diagnostic capacity. The techniques can be classified according to the frequency with which they are used: the *most common* are visual inspection (VI) and VI with magnification (VIM), the caries probe (CP), conventional X-rays (Rx) and digital X-rays (RxD); *less common* techniques (though still accessible to clinicians) are fiber-optic transillumination (FOTI and DiFOTI) and laser fluorescence (LF); and finally *unusual or experimental* techniques are those which presently are not generally used in clinical practice or which are still in the experimental phase – their use being confined to certain research settings. These latter techniques include the measurement of tissue electrical conductance, based on the reduction of electrical resistance or impedance that characterizes caried tissue (Pretty, 2006), using the electronic caries monitorization (ECM), while other methods are based on qualitative light-induced fluorescence (QLF) – which uses two types of fluorescence and generates images that can be filed for posterior comparison, with the capacity to determine whether the lesions are active or not. In turn, among the purely experimental techniques, mention should be made of optical coherence tomography (OCT), which generates images in the near-infrared region, and is able to detect incipient enamel caries *in vitro* (Ngaotheppitak et al., 2005).

2.1 Visual inspection (VI)

Visual inspection is the most widely used diagnostic method. VI has a long history, but is subjective and depends on the experience of the examiner (Pretty, 2006; Zandona & Zero, 2006). The diagnosis of a cavitated lesion poses no diagnostic difficulty of any kind; it is in the case of the so-called "hidden caries" where doubts arise, together with the impossibility of determining whether a dark fissure presents underlying caries or merely corresponds to surface staining. In their first stages, caries of grooves, pits and fissures appear as a milky or darkish stain indicating demineralization of the walls of the fissure and implying enamel opacity. In addition, there may be decoloration of the dentin through the enamel, as well as defects in the bottom or depth of the pit, which would confirm the diagnosis of dentin caries. Accordingly, clinical inspection is based on evaluation of the transparency changes of the enamel, loss of brightness, an opaque appearance, and integrity of the fissure (Thylstrup et al., 1994; Ekstrand et al., 1997). In order to appreciate these changes, the occlusal surfaces must be clean and dry during inspection of the grooves and fissures. Drying the enamel reduces the refraction index of the inter-rod spaces (from 1.33 in the case of humid or moist demineralized surfaces to 1.0 in the case of dry demineralized surfaces) – this making it possible to easily visualize the opaque appearance of enamel demineralization caused by the bacterial plaque acids (Kidd et al., 1993). We can also evaluate pigmentations, the presence or absence of soft tissues, or changes in enamel texture according to the degree of demineralization. According to some authors (Thylstrup et al., 1994), we are also able to establish whether the caries are active or inactive. The evaluation of these findings must be made following some classifying method or criterion capable of correlating the observed signs to the stage of the lesion. The system developed from the studies of Thylstrup in 1994 (Thylstrup et al., 1994) and posteriorly structured by Ekstrand in 1997 (Ekstrand et al., 1997) and modified in 1998 (Ekstrand et al., 1998) is one of the most widely used options. The criteria established by Ekstrand et al. (1997) are the following: 0 = no or slight change in enamel translucency after prolonged air drying; 1 = opacity or discoloration hardly visible on the wet surface, but distinctly visible after air drying; 2 = opacity or discoloration distinctly visible without air drying; 3 = localized enamel breakdown in opaque or discolored enamel and/or grayish discoloration from underlying dentin; and 4 = cavitation in opaque or discolored enamel exposing the dentin (Fig. 2). Other criteria have also been developed, however, such as those of Nyvad (Nyvad et al., 1999), the ICDAS (International Caries Detection and Assessment System (Pitts, 2004), the UniViSS (Universal Visual Scoring System for Caries Detection and Diagnosis) (Kuhnisch et al., 2009), or even the International Consensus Workshop on Caries Clinical Trials (ICW-CCT), where caries activity and inactivity are taken into consideration (Pitts & Stamm, 2004).

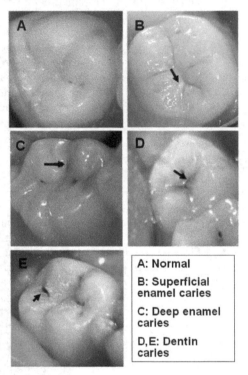

Fig. 2. Representative signs of caries in cracks and fissures, according to the Ekstrand criteria.

The sensitivity of visual inspection varies greatly depending on the literature source. Our review of the existing publications yielded values between 0.12 and 0.97. A sensitivity of 0.62 to 0.90 is common when there are visible cavities in the fissures. However, in hidden dentin caries, different studies (Lussi, 1993; Wenzel et al., 1991) have reported sensitivity values as low as 0.12. This low sensitivity is due to the fact that we cannot inspect beneath an apparently healthy enamel layer. Some authors (Ekstrand et al., 1997; Pereira et al., 2001) have obtained high sensitivity values that may be justified in part by elimination of a portion of the study sample due to validation problems or because of the presence of stained fissures. Application of the Ekstrand criteria tends to increase the sensitivity of the test both *in vitro* (Ekstrand et al., 1997; Tranæus et al., 2005) and *in vivo* (Angnes et al., 2005; Reis et al.,

2006). Some studies do not draw these conclusions, however (Heinrich-Weltzien et al., 2002). In effect, Lussi (Lussi et al., 2001) reported that visual inspection alone does not offer good sensitivity in detecting occlusal dentin caries. The width of the fissure also influences sensitivity; in this sense, a diagnosis is more difficult to establish in the presence of narrow fissures than in the case of wide fissures (Lussi, 1991). *In vivo* studies pose the inconvenience of incomplete sample validation, or the use of samples comprising third molars or premolars, with anatomical features different from those of the permanent first and second molars. Most studies indicate that visual inspection offers low-medium sensitivity and high specificity in the diagnosis of occlusal non-cavitated caries (Kidd et al., 1993; Wenzel et al., 1991; Reis et al., 2006; Heinrich-Weltzien et al., 2002) (Table 1).

AUTHOR	LEVEL	STUDY	SENSITIVITY	SPECIFICITY
Lussi 1993	dentin	*in vitro*	0.12	0.93
Ektrand 1997	dentin	*in vitro*	0.92 - 0.97	0.85 -0.93
Reis 2006	dentin	*in vitro*	0.69	0.88
Ashley 1998	enamel	*in vivo*	0.60	0.73
Angnes 2005	dentin	*in vivo*	0.75 / 0.68	0.84 / 0.81

Table 1. Sensitivity and specificity values for visual inspection.

In our studies (Abalos et al., 2009, 2011; Guerrero, 2011) of laser fluorescence, we obtained a sensitivity for visual inspection of over 0.70, in application to both enamel caries and dentin caries. In contrast to other authors, we achieved total validation of the sample of first and second molars *in vivo*, since we used teeth that were to be prepared for fixed prostheses. This afforded more realistic sensitivity and specificity values for the studied tests. However, in the case of VI, we consider that our results exceed those obtainable in the real life scenario, since as has been explained in our studies (Abalos et al., 2009, 2011; Guerrero, 2011), in our selection of the sample we aimed to secure a sufficient proportion of teeth that were clearly healthy or with enamel caries – a fact that may have influenced the recorded high sensitivity for VI. However, when using the criteria of Ekstrand (Ekstrand et al., 1997), with drying of the tooth (Tranæus et al., 2005; Ekstrand et al., 1997; Angnes et al., 2005; Reis et al., 2006), the sensitivity of the test increases. Many studies of VI have been published, and the results differ greatly according to the type of methodology used (Bader & Shugars, 2004). Despite this fact, VI is a technique that will continue to be used in routine clinical practice. However, rather than focusing on the true diagnostic performance of VI, which is clearly influenced by the examiner and the inaccessible depth of the fissures, future research should attempt to establish which tests are really useful, and to what extent, as coadjutants to visual inspection.

The mentioned moderate sensitivity is accompanied by high specificity (Table 1). In other words, while we must accept the probability of false-negative findings (Costa et al., 2008), the high specificity of the test and its important positive predictive value (PPV) (Guerrero, 2011) point to the advisability of opening all fissures with scores of 3 or 4 on the Ekstrand scale (Fig.2D,E). This is where the true usefulness of the test is found: when signs of caries are identified, caries may very well be present.

Regarding the reproducibility of the test, the studies that determine inter-examiner agreement or concordance (Lussi, 1991; Anttonen et al., 2003; Costa et al., 2008) report kappa

(k) values of >0.61 to >0.81. The reported intra-examiner reproducibility (Lussi, 1991; Anttonen et al., 2003; Costa et al., 2008) in turn yields k values of >0.41 to >0.81. This scale was developed by Landis and Koch (Landis & Koch, 1977), who scored the concordance values for the k index from <0 (no concordance) to 0–0.20 (insignificant or slight concordance), 0.21–0.40 (discrete concordance), 0.41–0.60 (moderate concordance), 0.61–0.80 (substantial concordance) and 0.81–1 (near-perfect concordance).

In sum, it is important for dentists to become familiarized with this exploration modality, without being too conditioned by superficially stained fissures that do not meet the specified criteria and which can lead to over-treatment. The prevalence of caries and the potential patient risk are important aspects that must be taken into account. A low caries prevalence with good molar hygiene and no bacterial plaque improve the reliability of the test, since there is a lesser probability of establishing an incorrect diagnosis. Visual inspection is the first method to be used in application to hidden dentin caries. In the case of a positive diagnosis, we should open the fissure and use a probe to explore the hardness of the dentin (Kidd et al., 1996). However, a negative diagnosis does not rule out the existence of caries, and other tests must be used together with VI in such situations – particularly in the presence of stained fissures.

2.2 Visual inspection with magnification (VIM)

Visual inspection with magnification (VIM) involves all the criteria and arguments defined for visual inspection (VI) without magnification. In the same way as with VI, the reported sensitivity data differ greatly, and can be as low as 0.20 (Lussi, 1993) – though accompanied by high specificity in most studies (Lussi, 1991). Magnification can improve the diagnostic performance of the test (Ekstrand et al., 1998; Lussi & Francescut, 2003). In this context, different studies have compared both methods (Lussi, 1993; Lussi, 1991; Lussi & Francescut, 2003), with the observation of superior sensitivity and specificity for VIM, though without reaching statistically significant differences versus VI. We obtained similar results, with a sensitivity rating for VIM (x2.6 magnification) of 0.76, versus 0.71 for VI (Guerrero, 2011). Our observed specificity (Guerrero, 2011) in turn is high, with a value of 0.84. In line with these results, Lussi (Lussi & Francescut, 2003) reported moderate sensitivity (0.65) and high specificity (0.96). Figure 3 simulates the view we would have of the occlusal surface of a lower second premolar without magnification (i.e., real size) and under x3.5 magnification. We can see that visual examination is easier with VIM; thus, although the literature reports no significant differences in performance between the two techniques, VIM is the preferred option, since it allows better appreciation of the possible signs of caries.

The importance of VI and VIM is attributable to their positive predictive value (PPV), which exceeds 90%(Guerrero 2011). In other words, when a positive diagnosis is established, caries is almost sure to be present. The same cannot be said of a negative diagnosis, however, since the negative predictive value (NPV) of the test is not so high. Therefore, we are unable to rule out the possibility of a false-negative diagnosis, since with this test it is often impossible to examine the depths of the fissures. In this sense, according to Lundberg (Lundberg et al., 2007), in the permanent first molars we observe a relationship between pit depth and bacterial colonization. Specifically, central pits are deeper and more varied in their morphology than less deeper mesial pits. There is an interesting correlation between central pits and colonization by *Streptococcus mutans*, and trapped organic material moreover may contribute to a faster evolution of hidden caries (Lundberg et al., 2007). In this sense, despite the use of magnification, visual inspection is far from being able to detect these etiopathogenic factors. In this sense, the visual diagnostic techniques require improvement or combination with other diagnostic methods in order to detect these early or incipient stages of caries. In conclusion, and in agreement with the studies of Forgie (Forgie et al., 2002) regarding the use of magnification in relation to other diagnostic techniques, VIM is the method of choice for the detection of occlusal non-cavitated caries, despite the limitations commented above.

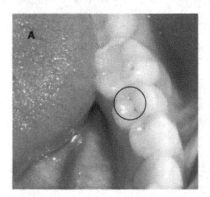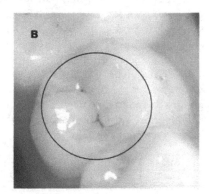

Fig. 3. Visual inspection of the occlusal surface of a second premolar (A: real size, and B:under x3.5 magnification).

2.3 Caries probing (CP) or tactile examination

Until recently, probe exploration formed part of the diagnostic routine in occlusal caries. Probe entrapment in the grooves and fissures helped in establishing the diagnosis. Although this technique is now contraindicated, some professionals continue to use caries probing (CP). The exploration probe has been evaluated as a diagnostic tool in many studies (Lussi, 1991; Lussi & Francescut, 2003). The sensitivity of CP in the detection of occlusal caries is 0.5-0.6 (Hamilton, 2005), though with high specificity values (Bader et al., 2002). The tip of the probe is unable to reach the bottom of the fissures, because of its thickness and the anatomy of the fissures. The probe tip size varies depending on the manufacturer. This lack of standardization of the tip size can make exploration difficult (Lussi, 1993). In addition, a number of studies (Lussi, 1991; Hibst et al., 2001; Hamilton, 2005) have demonstrated that a sharp-tipped probe can cause damage to recently erupted teeth and produce a cavity in a demineralized zone. As a result, the use of such instruments has been the subject of debate for years. Likewise, CP can transmit *Streptococcus mutans* from a contaminated fissure to a healthy fissure (Loesche et al., 1979). On the other hand, CP in combination with visual inspection (VI) does not improve the overall diagnostic performance of the exploration in application to caries of pits and fissures (Lussi, 1991; Lussi, 1993; McComb & Tam, 2001). Based on the above, the use of a round-tipped probe or periodontal probe alone would be justified for eliminating remnant material within the fissure before VI, and for evaluating the texture of the surface without penetrating the latter (Zandona & Zero, 2006; Ekstrand et al., 2005; Hamilton, 2005). Other applications would be contraindicated, however.

2.4 Conventional X-rays (Rx)

Clinical inspection is completed by radiological evaluation. Bitewing X-rays represent the technique of choice for diagnosing proximal surface caries, though they may also be useful for diagnosing occlusal dentin caries (Tranæus et al., 2005; Wenzel et al., 1992). At occlusal level, the X-rays register a tooth thickness beyond the proximal zone, and the lesions are masked by the healthy tissues for a longer period of time (Wenzel et al., 1992). For this reason, from the histological perspective, the lesion is more advanced than suggested by its radiological appearance – a fact that justifies the low sensitivity of the technique. In our studies, the observed sensitivity was 0.57 (Guerrero, 2011), i.e., many existing lesions are not detected. Nevertheless, once again, the specificity is very high. These results imply that negative X-ray findings cannot be taken to rule out dentin caries, though a positive X-ray diagnosis should be taken as an indication for opening the fissure and providing caries treatment. The reviewed *in vivo* and *in vitro* studies (Wenzel et al., 1992, Lussi, 1993; Angnes et al., 2005; Lussi et al., 2001; Ashley et al., 1998; Costa et al., 2008) point to low sensitivity and high specificity, in coincidence with our own results (Table 2). Only studies involving third molars report lesser specificity, possibly due to the difficulty of correctly obtaining X-ray projections in this zone.

AUTHOR	LEVEL	STUDY	SENSITIVITY	SPECIFICITY
Ashley 1998	enamel	*in vitro*	0.19	0.80
Wenzel 1990	enamel	*in vitro*	0.44	0.70
Ricketts 1997	dentin	*in vitro*	0.14	0.95
Ashley 1998	dentin	*in vitro*	0.24	0.89
Wenzel 1992	dentin	*in vitro*	0.48	0.81
Lussi 2001	dentin	*in vivo*	0.63	0.99
Heinrich 2002	dentin	*in vivo*	0.70	0.96
Angnes 2005	dentin	*in vivo*	0.0 - 0.06	0.98 - 0.96
Costa 2008	dentin	*in vivo*	0.26	0.94

Table 2. Sensitivity and specificity values for the X-ray diagnostic evaluation of occlusal caries.

The main difficulty of conventional X-ray exploration is the distinction between deep enamel and superficial dentin, due to superpositioning of the healthy vestibular and lingual enamel, which masks the radiotransparency, particularly in early-stage lesions. Carious lesions normally cannot be detected on X-rays until they have extended about 0.5 mm beyond the amelodentinal junction (Kidd et al., 1993). Even with this difficulty, however, *in vitro* studies point to acceptable correlation with the existing histological condition. In this context, Wenzel (Wenzel, 1998) suggested that the *in vitro* diagnostic performance may be better than in the actual clinical setting, i.e., the results obtained in the laboratory may be overestimated. However, other *in vitro* studies indicate that by the time occlusal caries have been identified on the X-rays, demineralization has already extended to the middle third of the dentinal layer, i.e., the deep dentin (Ricketts et al., 1997). Weerheijm (Weerheijm et al., 1992) reported that X-rays are not very effective for diagnosing incipient enamel caries, though the technique is very useful for diagnosing deeper lesions. In this context, conventional X-rays improve the diagnostic capacity of VI by 11%, and moreover help assess the extent of the lesion (Ekstrand et al., 1995).

Regarding the predictive value of the technique, our group (Guerrero, 2011) has recorded a PPV of 100%, suggesting that a positive diagnosis implies the existence of caries, since false-positive interpretations are very unlikely. In turn, we recorded a NPV of 59%, i.e., normal X-ray findings do not discard the possibility that an occlusal lesion may have invaded dentin. In relation to the inter-examiner reproducibility of the technique, the results are varied and range from kappa index (k) values of 0.39 (weak concordance) to 0.95 (near-perfect concordance) (Angnes et al., 2005; Costa et al., 2008; Cortes et al., 2000) – though most studies report substantial concordance values (0.61-0.80).

In sum, bitewing X-rays are an obligate diagnostic tool for proximal surface caries and represent a good adjunct in the diagnosis of occlusal caries. Considering that VI results in an important percentage of undetected clinical lesions (Wolwacz et al., 2004), particularly in adolescents (Wenzel et al., 1992), the bitewing X-rays must be carefully evaluated for possible lesions beneath the occlusal enamel. Figure 4 shows caries in dentin with a non-cavitated occlusal surface. However, a normal X-ray study does not rule out the presence of hidden dentin caries, in view of the low sensitivity and NPV of the technique.

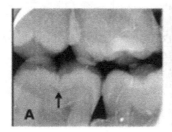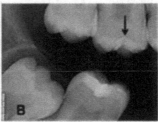

Fig. 4. Hidden dentin caries diagnosed from bitewing X-rays (A: dentin caries, B: early dentin caries)

2.5 Digital X-rays (RxD)

The application of digital X-rays (RxD) has gradually increased in dental practice, and the number of professionals who incorporate this technology to their personal practices is on the rise. RxD offer a number of advantages: the image is obtained immediately, with no need for development; the patient is exposed to a lesser radiation dose; and the images are examined using software that moreover allows them to be filed in electronic format, offering different forms of presentation and image measurements (Fig. 5).

In the same way as conventional X-rays, RxD offers low sensitivity and high specificity. We have recorded a sensitivity of 0.61 and a specificity of 0.96, i.e., practically without differences with respect to the conventional X-ray technique. The comparisons of these results with those found in the literature confirm the high specificity and limited sensitivity, though the reported sensitivity range is 0.30-0.70, versus 0.70-0.95 in the case of specificity (Table 3).

Regarding the comparison of both radiological techniques, some authors (Wenzel et al., 1992) consider that there are no differences between conventional X-rays and digital X-rays, in concordance with our own results. In contrast, other studies (Pretty, 2006; Lussi, 1993) have reported slightly greater sensitivity with RxD, and some investigators (McComb & Tam, 2001) consider that this technique improves diagnostic performance in early-stage caries. Further studies involving larger sample sizes are needed to confirm whether RxD improves diagnostic performance with respect to conventional X-rays. Similar considerations apply to VIM versus VI: it makes our work easier, diagnostic performance seems to be better, but analysis of the results fails to reveal statistically significant differences – the latter being taken to represent a difference of over 0.1 in sensitivity/specificity or a difference of over 10% in PPV/NPV.

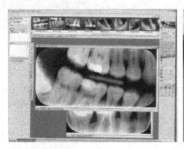 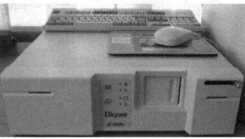

Fig. 5. Digital X-rays system (Digora Trophy Elitys)

AUTHOR	LEVEL	STUDY	SENSITIVITY	SPECIFICITY
Wenzel 1990	enamel	*in vitro*	0.31	0.72
Wenzel 1992	dentin	*in vitro*	0.71	0.85
Huysmans 1998	dentin	*in vitro*	0.52 - 0.60	0.91 – 0.95
Ashley 1998	dentin	*in vitro*	0.19	0.89
Wenzel 2008	dentin	*in vitro*	0.31	0.93

Table 3. Sensitivity and specificity values for the digital X-rays diagnostic evaluation of occlusal caries.

Regarding the predictive usefulness of the technique, in our study (Guerrero, 2011) the PPV of RxD was found to be 97%, i.e., a positive diagnostic reading implies the almost sure presence of caries. However, the same cannot be said when the diagnosis proves negative (i.e., indicative of a healthy tooth), since the proportion of false-negative results is high (NPV 60%).

2.6 Laser fluorescence (LF)

Laser fluorescence (LF) (Fig. 6) is less widely known and used by dental professionals, though it constitutes a necessary complement to the traditional methods. LF therefore deserves a more detailed description in this Chapter. Fluorescence occurs as a result of the interaction between electromagnetic radiation and tissue molecules. When light falls upon the surface of the tooth it penetrates a few millimeters into the tissue, and is reflected towards the tip of a device that measures the fluorescence by means of an electronic system. Two incremental ranges are observed in the fluorescence spectrum: one at 430-450 nm, related to demineralization of the tooth, and another at 590-650 nm, related to the presence of bacteria and their metabolites (Lundberg et al., 2007). Furthermore, there are other elements of organic and inorganic origin that can emit additional fluorescence and thus lead to error in the detection of caries: fluorosis, hypomineralization, bacterial plaque, calculus, proximal surface caries and other stains.

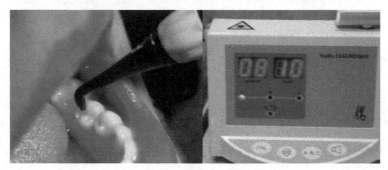

Fig. 6. Laser fluorescence device (DIAGNOdent, KaVo, Biberach, Germany)

The origin of the fluorescence is not fully clear (Pretty & Maupome, 2004; Tranæus et al., 2005), though it seems unlikely that apatite is responsible for the basal values associated with normal (healthy) enamel (Hibst et al., 2001). The explanation may be the result of the combination of the inorganic matrix with the absorption of organic molecules (Hibst & Paulus, 1999). During the formation of caries an increase in fluorescence is observed related to two processes: demineralization of the tooth, and bacteria with their metabolic products (porphyrin) (Pretty & Maupome, 2004; Tranæus et al., 2005). Most of the fluorescence is induced by the organic components (Tranæus et al., 2005; Hibst et al., 2001), rather than by crystal disintegration and transmission through scantly homogeneous enamel (Farah et al., 2008). This hypothesis is based on the fact that LF does not detect lesions caused in the laboratory with acids not produced as a result of bacterial activity (Pretty & Maupome, 2004). However, LF is able to detect early enamel lesions with a fluorescent stain (porphyrin TMPyP) (Mendes et al., 2006).

The results of the first *in vitro* studies with LF were promising, with high sensitivity and good reproducibility (Lussi et al., 1999). For dentin caries, many investigations have recorded sensitivity values in a very narrow range close to the highest values on the scale (0.79 – 1.0) (Bader & Shugars, 2004; Lussi et al., 1999). Few studies (Bader & Shugars, 2004) have described very low sensitivity (0.19 and 0.26) – such findings being attributable to subjectiveness and errors in the measurement technique during rotation of the instrument tip (Bader & Shugars, 2004; Reis et al., 2006). Although most studies report high sensitivity, the associated specificity is varied. The specificity values of LF in reference to dentin caries in permanent teeth ranges from 0.50 to 1.0 (Lussi et al., 2001; Pretty & Maupome, 2004; Başeren & Gokalp, 2003). Several studies (Bamzahim et al., 2002, 2000; Pereira et al., 2001) have reported near-perfect specificity for LF, thanks to the selection of those teeth with the highest LF readings (Bamzahim et al., 2002), while other authors explain the situation in terms of low sensitivity of the technique (Pereira et al., 2001). In the case of enamel caries the results are contradictory, with either moderate sensitivity ratings associated to high specificity values, or high sensitivity with moderate specificity (Table 4). High sensitivity is in agreement with the observations of previous *in vivo* studies, though without validation based on fissurotomy (Anttonen et al., 2003; Lussi & Francescut, 2003). The above considerations are also consistent with other studies involving histological validation and measurement of third molars (Reis et al., 2006), and with *in vitro* investigations involving third molars stored at -20°C (Lussi & Hellwig, 2006). In our study (Abalos et al., 2011), high sensitivity was accompanied by limited specificity (0.63) which, although coinciding with the findings of other authors (Bader & Shugars, 2004; Reis et al., 2006) is lower than in others studies (Lussi et al., 2000; Baseren & Gokalp, 2003; Anttonen et al., 2003; Lussi & Hellwig, 2006). Low specificity could be partially due to the fact that we did not eliminate teeth with the presence of brown or dark spots on fissures from the study sample. This low specificity at D_1 level (healthy/enamel caries) is less important than at D_3 level (enamel caries/dentin caries), where the proportion of false-positive readings can have negative consequences, since it can lead to over-treatment. Table 4 summarizes the results of some representative studies in relation to sensitivity and specificity, though for reasons that will be addressed below, the findings of our investigations (Abalos et al., 2009; 2011) may actually be closest to the true situation.

AUTHOR	LEVEL	STUDY	SENSITIVITY	SPECIFICITY
Lussi 2001	enamel	*in vitro*	0.38 - 0.95	0.24 - 0.95
Stookey 2001	enamel	*in vitro*	0.42 - 0.87	0.72 – 0.95
Abalos 2011	enamel	*in vivo*	0.97	0.63
Lussi 1999	dentin	*in vitro*	0.76 – 0.84	0.79 – 0.87
Hibst 2001	dentin	*in vitro*	0.92	0.86
Stookey 2001	dentin	*in vitro*	0.76 – 0.84	0.79 – 1.00
Heinrich 2003	dentin	*in vitro*	0.93 – 0.99	0.13 – 0.63
Reis 2006	dentin	*in vitro*	0.71 - 0.78	0.57 - 0.63
Lussi 2001	dentin	*in vivo*	0.92	0.86
Agnes 2005	dentin	*in vivo*	0.68 - 0.81	0.56 - 0.54
Reis 2006	dentin	*in vivo*	0.80 - 0.75	0.43 - 0.52
Abalos 2009	dentin	*in vivo*	0.89	0.75

Table 4. Sensitivity and specificity of laser fluorescence in the diagnosis of occlusal non-cavitated caries.

Most studies evaluating LF have been carried out *in vitro* (Tranæus et al., 2005; Stookey & Gonzalez-Cabezas, 2001; Hibst et al., 2001; Bader & Shugars, 2004; Lussi et al., 1999), though there are also a number of *in vivo* studies (Anttonen et al., 2003; Angnes et al., 2005; Heinrich-Weltzien et al., 2003; Lussi et al., 2001; Reis et al., 2006; Abalos et al., 2009; Abalos et al., 2011). The results of *in vitro* studies cannot be extrapolated to *in vivo* conditions, and the limitations of these studies are know. The way in which the teeth are preserved, or the changes in their organic content after extraction, are the main factors inducing alterations in dental tissue fluorescence. The mentioned organic matrix begins to degrade in the second week of preservation of the tooth. When teeth are preserved in formalin, thymol or chlorine (Francescut et al., 2006), the fluorescence value in the occlusal surface decreases rapidly in the first 5 months (Lussi & Francescut, 2003). This in turn implies a drop in the LF values (Lussi et al., 1999) and favors the obtainment of high specificity results. On the other hand, *in vitro* studies make no mention of the age and origin of the samples. *In vivo* studies also pose limitations; in effect, in order to ensure total sample validation, these studies are made in third molars or premolars selected for extraction due to surgical or orthodontic indications. The occlusal anatomy in this case differs from that of the permanent first and second premolars, as a result of which the results must be viewed with caution (Heinrich-Weltzien et al., 2003). In the case of *in vivo* studies conducted in permanent first and second molars, the teeth presumed to be healthy or with enamel caries cannot be validated due to ethical reasons. The authors must assume the standard, without being able to confirm or discard the presence of caries via fissurotomy. As a result, it is not possible to detect the existence of false-negative readings, which are frequent in the visual inspection-based diagnostic procedure used for sample selection. Two options are available in this situation: elimination of the non-validated teeth, whereby the prevalence will be almost 100%, or assumption of the possible existence of false-negative readings in the gold standard. In both cases, the calculations are not precise, and the results must be examined with caution – as pointed out in the literature (Lussi et al., 2001; Heinrich-Weltzien et al., 2003). Only our *in vivo* studies (Abalos et al., 2009; 2011; Guerrero, 2011) involve permanent first and second molars with total sample validation, since the category of healthy teeth or teeth with enamel caries could be validated. The molars were to serve as abutments for fixed prostheses, and could be validated via fissurotomy before being worked upon. An alternative for the use of an imperfect reference standard method is mathematical correction of the values of sensitivity and specificity (Brenner, 1996). This adjustment could approximate the performance obtained in the studies to the actual performance of the methods, increasing the external validity of the study. This procedure has been employed by Matos (2011) for the first time in studies of caries detection. Another alternative to *in vivo* evaluations is the conduction of *in vitro* studies, but with frozen teeth (Lussi & Hellwig, 2006), which allows clinical extrapolation of the results. Other limitations in LF studies are represented by plaque or organic material remains, stains, the degree of tooth dehydration, composite fillings or traces of polishing paste – all of which can affect the LF readings, since they are sources of fluorescence and can therefore give rise to false-positive results. In addition, other factors (Abalos & Jiménez-Planas, 2011) inherent to the tooth such as age, the degree of maturation, and the depth of the pits can influence the measurements obtained (Lundberg et al., 2007).

The variation in LF readings found by our group is considerable (Abalos et al., 2009; 2011), in the same way as in other clinical studies (Anttonen et al., 2003; Lussi et al., 2001). However, the mean values show a gradient through the different categories of lesion extent (D_0: healthy; D_{1+2}: enamel caries; D_{3+4}: dentin caries) that increases as caries progresses (Lussi et al., 2001). This gradient is observed in both *in vitro* (Başeren & Gokalp, 2003) and in *in vivo* studies (Astvaldsdottir et al., 2004; Anttonen et al., 2003; Heinrich-Weltzien et al., 2003; Lussi et al., 2001; Heinrich-Weltzien et al., 2002), and in both permanent teeth (Astvaldsdottir et al., 2004; Heinrich-Weltzien et al., 2003; Lussi et al., 2001; Heinrich-Weltzien et al., 2002) and temporary teeth (Anttonen et al., 2003; Lussi & Francescut, 2003) – though the values are lower in the case of the primary dentition. In our investigations (Abalos et al., 2009; 2011) LF was seen to be able to distinguish between enamel caries and dentin caries (Abalos et al., 2009), though without being able to discriminate between healthy teeth and teeth with enamel caries (Abalos et al., 2011). The explanation for this latter observation is that the initial enamel lesion does not induce a significant increase in fluorescence when compared with healthy enamel. Likewise, Lussi in 1999 (Lussi et al., 1999) reported that LF does not seem very adequate for detecting minor changes in the enamel. Some studies (Astvaldsdottir et al., 2004) have reported a weak correlation between the LF readings and the depth of the lesion, though this does not suffice to view LF as a method for determining depth. In other words, while LF appears to be able to establish when lesions invade one tissue or other, it is not useful for discriminating depth within one same tissue, whether enamel or dentin (Lussi et al., 2001; Başeren & Gokalp, 2003).

At present, the cutoff values are based on those established by Lussi in 2001 in the context of a clinical study (Lussi et al., 2001), with standardization as follows: 0-13 for healthy teeth, 14-20 for enamel caries, and >20 for dentin caries. The results of our group are in concordance with these cutoff values (Abalos et al., 2009; 2011), in the same way as in other clinical studies . Our values (Abalos et al., 2011) for healthy first and second molars assessed *in vivo* range between 0 and 14. Values below 10 in all cases corresponded to healthy fissures. The only previous studies (Başeren & Gokalp, 2003; Sheehy et al., 2001) made to determine the limits in healthy enamel have been conducted *in vitro* (Başeren & Gokalp, 2003) or *in vivo* in third molars (Sheehy et al., 2001), with histological validation. Laser fluorescence readings of >14 in turn can be indicative of enamel caries, while readings of ≥ 20 can mean dentin caries, though without necessarily implying operative intervention. As advised by Lussi (Lussi et al., 2001), in patients with low caries risk, fissure aperture should be indicated at LF readings of ≥ 30.

In contrast to the previously examined techniques, LF is more sensitive than specific, and so implies a greater number of false-positive readings. These readings are normally explained by fluorescence sources unrelated to caries – stained fissures being the main problem facing diagnosis with LF (Angnes et al., 2005; Heinrich-Weltzien et al., 2003) (Fig. 7). The stains contribute an added fluorescence signal that increases the measurement values obtained (Côrtes et al., 2003) by between 5-7 units (Heinrich-Weltzien et al., 2003; Sheehy et al., 2001), and represent a frequent cause of overestimation (Sheehy et al., 2001) and of lessened performance of the test. This must be taken into account in order to adjust or modify the cutoff value. When conducting their studies, investigators must specify the percentage of stained fissures in order to allow improved comparison of the results. In our studies (Abalos et al., 2009; 2011; Guerrero 2011) the percentage was approximately 25%. Cases of under-estimation are rare, and any such situations are attributable to a poor measurement technique and failure to have rotated the instrument tip in all directions.

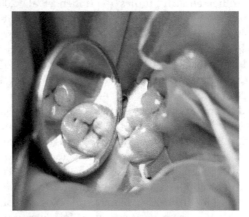

Fig. 7. Stained fissure complicating laser fluorescence (LF) diagnosis.

Receiver operating characteristic (ROC) curves take sensitivity and specificity into account for all the cutoff points, thereby reflecting the global diagnostic capacity of the technique. This analysis also offers the average validity of the method used. Taking Az to represent the area under the ROC curve, Az = 1 would represent perfect diagnostic accuracy. In general, a value of Az ≥ 0.80 is regarded as acceptable, and would mean that the probability of effectively identifying caries is 80%. ROC analysis shows LF to be a good diagnostic technique in application to enamel caries, with Az = 0.803 (Abalos et al., 2011). These results are somewhat inferior to those reported by other investigators (Stookey & Gonzalez-Cabezas, 2001). For dentin caries Az = 0.85, reflecting good diagnostic reliability. These findings coincide with those of some *in vivo* investigations (Heinrich-Weltzien et al., 2003), but exceed the values of 0.64–0.69 described by other *in vivo / in vitro* studies (Angnes et al., 2005), with histological validation in reference to third molars.

Comparison of the different diagnostic tests can be based on their respective sensitivity and specificity performances, which reflect the comparative reliability of each technique. The NPV value for occlusal dentin caries was 87%, with a PPV value of 79%. The concepts of sensitivity and specificity therefore allow us to assess the validity of a given diagnostic test. Both sensitivity and specificity offer information on the probability of obtaining a concrete result or reading (positive or negative), according to the true condition of the patient in relation to the disease. However, when a patient is subjected to a test, the dentist lacks prior information on the true diagnosis, and the question is actually posed from a reverse perspective: in the event of a positive or negative test result, what is the probability that the patient is actually ill or healthy? Thus, the predictive values complement the information provided by sensitivity and specificity. The results obtained reflect a high NPV and an acceptable PPV. Therefore, LF is a complement to those tests offering high specificity and a high PPV. LF is a coadjuvant to VI, and the use of both techniques combined increases the number of correctly diagnosed lesions.

2.7 Qualitative light-induced fluorescence (QLF)

Qualitative light-induced fluorescence (QLF) is used for the detection and quantification of early-stage caries (Pretty, 2006; McComb & Tam, 2001) and for monitoring demineralization or remineralization of smooth surface lesions (Verdonschot & van der Veen, 2002; Heinrich-Weltzien et al., 2005). The tooth is illuminated by the diffuse blue-green light beam of an argon laser at a wavelength of 488 nm (Tranæus et al., 2005; McComb & Tam, 2001). It can also be illuminated by a xenon microdischarge arc lamp and optic fiber system generating blue light at a wavelength of 370 nm (Pretty, 2006), with conduction by a liquid guide. The images are obtained in a dimmed environment using a portable intraoral video camera, with software processing. These images can be used to calculate lesion size, depth and volume (Tranæus et al., 2005; Zandona & Zero, 2006). The demineralized areas appear as dark zones, since radiation of the carious lesion is lower than that of the healthy enamel (Tranæus et al., 2005). The intensity of the emitted light is correlated to mineral loss and can be quantified (Verdonschot & van der Veen, 2002).

QLF is sensitive and reproducible in quantifying smooth surface caries, though it does not discriminate between lesions confined to the enamel layer and dentin caries (McComb & Tam, 2001). The applicability of this technique appears to be limited by lesion depth (McComb & Tam, 2001) – QLF being effective up to 400 µm in depth, but not beyond. The possibility of adapting the technique to the diagnosis of occlusal caries is under investigation, though few clinical studies have been made to date (Weerheijm et al., 1992; McComb & Tam, 2001). Table 5 shows the sensitivity and specificity data of *in vitro* studies on QLF in application to occlusal dentin caries. This diagnostic technique can be affected by the degree of humidity or dryness of the fissures, their stains and morphology and does not appear to distinguish between caries and hypoplasia.

AUTHOR	LEVEL	STUDY	SENSITIVITY	SPECIFICITY
Stookey 2001	Dentin	*in vitro*	0.49	0.67
Zandona 2006	Dentin	*in vitro*	0.61	0.59
Pretty 2004	Dentin	*in vitro*	0.77	0.67
McComb 2001	Dentin	*in vitro*	0.72-0.76	0.79-0.81

Table 5. Sensitivity and specificity of QLF in the diagnosis of hidden dentin caries.

2.8 Fiber-optic transillumination (FOTI)

Fiber-optic transillumination (FOTI) (Fig. 8) is a qualitative technique introduced in the 1970s. It is based on light transmission through an optic fiber; as the light falls upon the tooth surface, it spreads through the healthy dental tissue. In this context, caried tissue is characterized by an increased organic component, with alteration of the homogeneity of the inorganic component – thereby resulting in a loss of light transmission capacity.

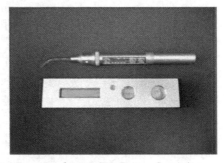

Fig. 8. Fiber-optic transillumination device (DioPower Lamp)

FOTI has been used fundamentally for identifying proximal surface caries (Cortes et al., 2000;), with high specificity and a broader range of sensitivity values (Tranæus et al., 2005). The technique is of great help in diagnosing cracked tooth syndrome (Fig. 9). However, it is little used for diagnosing hidden dentin caries, where moreover few studies have assessed its diagnostic performance, precision and reproducibility.

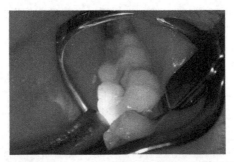

Fig. 9. Cracked tooth syndrome diagnosed by fiber-optic transillumination (FOTI).

FOTI is more specific than sensitive. Table 6 reports the validity of the test in different *in vitro* studies referred to occlusal caries. In an *in vivo* study with full sample validation, our group (Guerrero, 2011) has recorded a sensitivity of 0.47 and a specificity of 1.0. These data are in line with those reported by other *in vitro* studies (Ashley et al., 1998; Cortes et al., 2000).

AUTHOR	LEVEL	STUDY	SENSITIVITY	SPECIFICITY
Cortes 2000	enamel	*in vitro*	0.74 - 1	0.23 – 0.85
Ashley 1998	enamel	*in vitro*	0.21	0.95
Cortes 2000	dentin	*in vitro*	0.74	0.85
Ashley 1998	dentin	*in vitro*	0.14	0.95

Table 6. Sensitivity and specificity of FOTI in the diagnosis of occlusal non-cavitated caries.

As a coadjutant to visual inspection, FOTI can offer an alternative to X-rays in situations where patient irradiation is not possible. It is therefore interesting to compare both methods. In reference to occlusal caries, some authors (Wenzel et al., 1992) consider transillumination to offer better performance than conventional X-rays in detecting early-stage dentin caries. Cortés (Cortes et al., 2000), in an *in vitro* study, reported greater sensitivity than specificity for FOTI, and superior performance with respect to X-rays, though in application to the diagnosis of enamel caries. Once caries has progressed to the dentin, FOTI proved to be significantly inferior to conventional X-rays (Guerrero, 2011). Regarding the predictive usefulness of the technique, we recorded a NPV of 54% and a PPV of 100%, without false-positive readings (Guerrero, 2011).

However, the fact that FOTI is not routinely used by dental professionals, is not recommended as a technique of choice, and is moreover supported by limited research indicates that the inconveniences which we have observed (Guerrero, 2011) – involving a large proportion of false-negative results – are probably coincident with those of other authors who have studied this technique. The main advantage of FOTI is its optimum PPV performance, which means that any positive reading is almost certainly indicative of an existing lesion.

Digitalization may represent a step forward in transillumination diagnosis. Digital FOTI (DIFOTI) makes use of the digitalized image of a tooth during transillumination, which is analyzed using specific software (Trandæus et al., 2005). The images can be filed, reproduced and studied by different examiners, and may serve to monitor the lesion. Interpretation of the image is where problems are found, however, since the results are not directly quantified by the technique. According to some authors (Pretty & Maupome, 2004; Pretty, 2006), the caried areas can be detected in their early stages with DIFOTI, appearing as dark areas. The results may be superior to those afforded by radiography (Pretty & Maupome, 2004; Pretty, 2006), though further studies are needed in order to confirm this possibility.

To summarize, FOTI in combination with visual inspection may be useful for determining occlusal caries depth, though further *in vivo* studies are needed. While in wait of such studies, we consider that transillumination should not be used for diagnosing hidden dentin caries, due to the low sensitivity of the technique and its poorer results compared with X-rays. However, FOTI in combination with VI should be taken into consideration in those cases where X-rays cannot be obtained.

2.9 Electronic caries monitorization (ECM)

Electronic caries monitorization (ECM) is based on the high electrical conduction resistance of the hard dental tissues. Enamel is a poor electrical conductor though caried enamel shows increased conductance versus intact enamel (Loesche et al., 1979). Demineralized enamel becomes more porous, fills with ion-containing fluid and minerals from saliva, and therefore exhibits increased electrical conductance (McComb & Tam, 2001).

Two devices have been developed, with tips designed for application to the occlusal surface and for measuring electrical conductance in pits or fissures (Zandona & Zero, 2006). The Electronic Caries Monitor (LODE, Groningen, the Netherlands), in the same way as its predecessor (Vanguard, Electronic Caries Detector, Massachusetts Manufacturing Cooperation Cambridge, MA, USA), was developed for diagnosing occlusal surface caries, and allows the identification of early-stage demineralization lesions. The sensitivity performance in application to permanent premolars and molars varies from 0.67 to 0.96, with specificity values of between 0.71 and 0.98 (Tranæus et al., 2005; Pereira et al., 2001; Lussi et al., 1999). The different reviews of ECM describe similar results, with sensitivity values referred to dentin lesions of 0.58 to 0.97 and specificity values between 0.56 and 0.94. One of the reasons for this range of results may be due to the differences in the way in which the technique is used. The degree of dental tissue hydration may also exert an influence, in the same way as enamel maturation and temperature variations (Tranæus et al., 2005; Pretty, 2006). Table 7 shows the sensitivity and specificity performances recorded from *in vitro* and *in vivo* studies with ECM applied to occlusal caries.

AUTHOR	LEVEL	STUDY	SENSITIVITY	SPECIFICITY
Ashley 1998	enamel	*in vitro*	0.65	0.73
Ekstrand 1997	enamel	*in vivo*	0.63	0.73
Lussi 1999	dentin	*in vitro*	0.58 - 0.92	0.76 - 0.94

Table 7. Sensitivity and specificity of ECM in the diagnosis of occlusal non-cavitated caries.

2.10 Conclusions of the diagnostic tests

Modern dental practice needs diagnostic methods to diagnose caries in the early stages of the disease, and research efforts must focus on satisfying this need. The traditional diagnostic techniques offer high specificity, but with the possibility of false-negative results due to dentin caries. Laser fluorescence (LF) shows high sensitivity, and is able to identify hidden dentin caries in situations where visual inspection (VI) and X-rays are unable to detect the lesions. However, because of its lesser specificity and the low current prevalence of caries in the industrialized world, LF should be used as a coadjutant to VI in diagnosing hidden dentin caries. It has been estimated that an additional 30-50% of non-cavitated occlusal caries can be detected in the early stages with LF. Bitewing X-rays represent a complement to VI, but is only able to detect the lesion once it has advanced in the dentinal tissue. As a result, different studies (Anttonen et al., 2003; Ricketts et al., 1997) consider LF to be more effective than bitewing X-rays as an adjunct to VI in diagnosing occlusal caries.

Based on the results obtained, the combination of LF and VI appears as an interesting option. In effect, the two techniques complement each other, securing superior overall performance, since one (LF) is more sensitive than specific, while the other (VI) is more specific than sensitive. When interpreting the results of diagnostic tests, a negative diagnostic result is sometimes more valuable than a positive diagnostic reading. This can be explained as follows: although clinicians seek values from which caries can be diagnosed, the opposite sometimes apply. In effect, we have observed that LF readings of under 10 will never indicate an actual caried tooth, and LF readings of under 20 in stained fissures or cracks will never indicate or correspond to dentin caries. Thus, a first conclusion could be that in the case of a doubtful VI result with LF values of under 10 involving adequate instrument tip rotation, we must assume that the tissue is healthy, in the same way that LF readings of under 20 in stained fissures do not correspond to dentin caries. LF readings of 10-20 with normal VI findings are indicative of healthy tissue, particularly in the presence of some fissure staining. However, in the differential diagnosis between healthy tissue and enamel caries (D_0-D_1), over-estimation of the lesion is not particularly important, since the treatment involved is of a preventive nature. LF is a help in VI, particularly when the findings of the latter are not clear and a diagnosis cannot be established. LF moreover acquires an added diagnostic value when its readings are low in stained fissures or high in unstained fissures. All teeth with readings above 14 must be subjected to preventive measures and monitorization or control. In turn, LF readings of over 20 can imply that the lesion has reached the dentin, though the experience of the operator and the patient risk factors must always be taken into account. The most important conclusions of this Chapter, based on our investigations (Abalos et al., 2009; 2011; Guerrero, 2011), can be listed as follows:

1. Visual inspection, with or without magnification, is the method of choice for diagnosing non-cavitated caries. For adequate diagnostic performance, use must be made of the Ekstrand criteria, combining VI with other techniques such as LF. Visual inspection is more specific than sensitive, and so a positive diagnosis requires fissure aperture, while a negative diagnostic interpretation is inconclusive and required periodic revisions.

2. Conventional or digital X-rays constitute a necessary complementary technique. Its high specificity means that in the case of a positive diagnosis, fissure aperture should be carried out, and it can be used to assess the extent of the lesion. X-rays are not useful for the diagnosis of very early stage lesions.

3. Laser fluorescence is a useful technique that serves as an adjunct or complement to visual inspection, offering high sensitivity and acceptable specificity. LF readings of under 10 are indicative of a healthy tooth, while readings of over 20 may indicate dentin invasion – though the definitive interpretation must be made in combination with visual inspection. In turn, readings of 10-20 indicate that lesion monitorization is required. LF is unable to establish the depth of the lesion within the tissue (either enamel or dentin). Low readings in stained fissures rule out dentin caries.

4. Probe exploration is not recommended for diagnosing non-cavitated caries. Fiber-optic transillumination (FOTI) is not a method of choice, since it is scantly sensitive – though it may serve as a complementary technique when X-rays cannot be obtained.

5. The combination of exploratory techniques, together with technical and scientific knowledge, are essential for establishing a correct diagnosis of non-cavitated caries. The individual patient factors must be taken into account in order to indicate fissure aperture or periodic revisions or controls.

3. Intervention protocol

Based on the results obtained, and in the context of the diagnostic techniques that are accessible to dental surgeons, we recommend the following protocol:

→ Positive X-ray or FOTI findings............................. Dentin caries

→ Visual inspection (better under magnification):
   - **Ekstrand score 0:**   - If LF < 14 ....No Caries
                              - If LF 15-20 .... Monitorization enamel
                                 *Stained fissure............... No caries
                              - If LF > 20 ....Monitorization dentin

→ Visual inspection (better under magnification):
   - **Ekstrand score 1-2:** - If LF < 10............................No Caries
                              - If LF 10-20 .... Enamel caries
                              - If LF > 20 ....Monitorization dentin
                                 *Stained fissure ....Monitorization enamel

→ Visual inspection (better under magnification):
   - **Ekstrand score 3-4:** - If LF < 20............................2nd measure rotating tip
                                 *2nd LF < 20..................Enamel caries
                              - If LF > 20 ....Dentin caries
                                 *Stained fissure ....Fissure aperture

4. Treatment

The present Chapter focuses on techniques applicable to the diagnosis of hidden dentin caries. However, as a complement to the measures recommended in the above intervention protocol, we will outline the therapeutic approach applicable to each diagnosis.

4.1 Fissure aperture

Fissure aperture applies when we believe but cannot fully confirm that dentin caries exists. A fissurotomy drill is used to open the fissure, crack or pit until reaching the dentin. A fine-tipped probe is then used to check dentin hardness, and if there are no carious lesions, crack sealant is applied. In contrast, if caries is identified, the lesion is eliminated, followed by filling with composite resin or silver amalgam.

4.2 Enamel monitorization

In this case the doubt is whether enamel caries exists or not. Bacterial plaque control is indicated in these situations, based on oral and dental hygiene measures and topical fluor application. If the suspicion of caries results from high LF readings with normal VI findings, monitorization fundamentally should be carried out with LF. The detection of positive VI signs or increased LF readings during follow-up, potentially indicative of lesion progression, requires fissure aperture.

If caries is suspected on the basis of the VI findings, with normal LF results, the subsequent controls should be centered on VI. The detection of an increase in positive VI signs or increased LF readings during follow-up, potentially indicative of dentin involvement, requires fissure aperture.

4.3 Enamel caries

Treatment should distinguish between active and inactive lesions, since such a distinction is important in management terms. The development of techniques for differentiating between active and inactive lesions is thus seen as a necessity, since very few studies in this field have been published to date (Bader & Shugars, 2004). The general clinician experiences great difficulty in distinguishing between these lesions (Ekstrand et al., 2005). When the band and plaque are removed, the clinical features of the active lesion have been recorded as a dull/opaque white area, which is said to be rough when a probe is moved across the surface. Accordingly, the signs for establishing a differentiation are: a) Whether the lesion was dull/matt or shiny/glossy; and b) The tactile sensation of the lesion to a ball-ended probe run gently across the surface was recorded as smooth or rough to the probe.

According to some studies (Pretty, 2006), laser fluorescence is able to establish differences between the readings corresponding to active and inactive enamel caries in permanent molars. In this sense, LF would be able to serve in monitoring the lesion. However, other studies (Toraman et al., 2008) consider that the technique does not register the changes that occur during remineralization and caries development arrest, and cannot serve for monitorization purposes.

Following improved oral hygiene, the lesion is no longer active, and there may be remineralization within the lesion and abrasion of the eroded surface enamel during oral hygiene procedures and normal function. This leads to a surface which feels smooth when a probe is gently run across it, and which appears shinier (Thylstrup et al., 1994). Once inactive, monitoring of the lesion should continue. Persistent activity is indicative of the need for fissure aperture and the placement of crack sealant.

4.4 Dentin monitorization

Laser fluorescence readings of under 20 in the presence of positive visual inspection findings are suggestive of dentin caries. Fissure aperture would be indicated with LF readings of over 20.

4.5 Dentin caries

Enamel aperture with a diamond drill, followed by elimination of the caried dentin with adequate instruments, is indicated in the case of dentin caries. Filling with resin composites or silver amalgam should follow. Ceramic incrustations may be considered in the case of important tooth involvement.

Both the described intervention protocol and the specified treatments cannot encompass all the possible clinical situations. Likewise, they cannot replace clinician experience and the global vision afforded by all the diagnostic techniques, the tooth and oral conditions, and even the individual conditions of each patient. However, the information provided may serve to establish bases and guidelines for intervention and recommendations fundamented on experience and research.

5. References

Abalos, C. Herrera, M. Jimenez-Planas, A. Llamas, R. (2009). Performance of laser fluorescence for detection of occlusal dentinal caries lesions in permanent molars: an in vivo study with total validation of the sample. *Caries Res,* Vol.43, No.2, PP.137-141, ISSN 0008-6568.

Abalos, C. Jiménez-Planas, A. (2011) La Láser-Fluorescencia en el diagnóstico temprano de la caries no cavitada. *Dentum,* Vol.11, No.1, pp.20-23, ISNN 1575-6157.

Abalos, C. Mendoza, A. Jiménez-Planas, A. Guerrero, A. Chaparro, A. García-Godoy, F. (2012) Clinical detection of enamel caries by laser fluorescence. *Am J Dent,* (In press), ISSN 0894-8275.

Angnes, V. Angnes, G. Batisttella, M. Grande, RH. Loguercio, AD. Reis, A. (2005) Clinical effectiveness of laser fluorescence, visual inspection and radiography in the detection of occlusal caries. *Caries Res,* Vol.39, No.6, pp.490-495, ISSN 0008-6568.

Anttonen, V. Seppa, L. Hausen, H. (2003) Clinical study of the use of the laser fluorescence device DIAGNOdent for detection of occlusal caries in children. *Caries Res,* Vol.37, No.1, pp.17-23, ISSN 0008-6568.

Ashley, PF. Blinkhorn, AS. Davies, RM. (1998). Occlusal caries diagnosis: an in vitro histological validation of the Electronic Caries Monitor (ECM) and other methods. *J Dent,* Vol.26, No.2, pp.83-88, ISSN 0300-5712.

Astvaldsdottir, A. Holbrook, WP. Tranaeus, S. (2004). Consistency of Diagnodent instruments for clinical assement of fissure caries. *Act Odon Scand,* Vol.62, No.4, pp.193-198, ISSN 0001-6357.

Bader, JD. Shugars, DA. Bonito, AJ. (2002). A systematic review of the performance of methods for identifying carious lesions. *J Public Health Dent,* Vol.62, No.4, pp201-213, ISSN 0022-4006.

Bader. JD, Shugars, DA. (2004). A systematic review of the performance of a laser fluorescence device for detecting caries. *J Am Dent Assoc,* Vol.135, No.10, pp.1413-1426, ISSN 0002-8177.

Bagramian, RA. Garcia-Godoy, F. Volpe, AR. (2009). The global increase in dental caries. A pending public health crisis. *Am J Dent,* Vol.22, pp.3-8, ISSN 0894-8275.

Bamzahim, M. Shi, X-. Angmar-Mansson, B. (2002). Occlusal caries detection and quantification by DIAGNOdent and Electronic Caries Monitor: In vitro comparison. *Acta Odontologica Scandinavica,* Vol.60, No.6, pp.360-364, ISSN 0001-6357.

Baseren, NM. Gokalp, S. (2003). Validity of a laser fluorescence system (DIAGNOdent) for detection of occlusal caries in third molars: An in vitro study. *Journal of Oral Rehabilitation,* Vol.30, No.12, pp.1190-1194, ISSN 0305-182X.

Bonilla, V. (1998). Estudio comparativo del diagnóstico "in vivo" de la caries de superficie proximal con radiografía convencional y laservisiografía en 145 dientes del sector posterior. *Ph.Thesis,* University of Seville.

Brännstrom, M. Gola, G. Nordenvall, Kj. Torstenson, B. (1980). Invasion of microorganisms and some structural changes in incipient enamel caries. *Caries Res,* Vol.14, pp.276-84, ISSN 0008-6568.

Brenner, H. (1996). Correcting for exposure misclassification using an alloyed gold standard. *Epidemiology,* Vol.7, pp.406–410, ISNN 1044-3983.

Cortes, DF. Ekstrand, KR. Elias-Boneta, AR. Ellwood, RP. (2000). An in vitro comparison of the ability of fibre-optic transillumination, visual inspection and radiographs to detect occlusal caries and evaluate lesion depth. *Caries Res*, Vol.34, No.6, pp.443-447, ISSN 0008-6568.

Costa, AM. Paula, LM. Bezerra, AC. (2008). Use of Diagnodent for diagnosis of non-cavitated occlusal dentin caries. *J Appl Oral Sci*, Vol.16, No.1, pp.18-23, ISSN 1678-7757.

Ekstrand, KR. Kuzmina, I. Bjorndal, L. Thylstrup, A. (1995). Relationship between external and histologic features of progressive stages of caries in the occlusal fossa. *Caries Res*, Vol.29, No.4, pp.243-250, ISSN 0008-6568.

Ekstrand, KR. Ricketts, DN. Kidd, EA. (1997). Reproducibility and accuracy of three methods for assessment of demineralization depth of the occlusal surface: an in vitro examination. *Caries Res*, Vol.31, No.3, pp.224-231, ISSN 0008-6568.

Ekstrand, KR. Ricketts, DN. Kidd, EA. Qvist, V. Schou, S. (1998). Detection, diagnosing, monitoring and logical treatment of occlusal caries in relation to lesion activity and severity: an in vivo examination with histological validation. *Caries Res*, Vol.32, No.4, pp.247-254, ISSN 0008-6568.

Ekstrand, KR. Ricketts, DN. Longbottom, C. Pitts, NB. (2005). Visual and tactile assessment of arrested initial enamel carious lesions: an in vivo pilot study. *Caries Res*, Vol.39, No.3, pp.173-177, ISSN 0008-6568.

Farah, RA. Drummond, BK. Swain, MV. (2008). Williams S. Relationship between laser fluorescence and enamel hypomineralisation. *J Dent*, Vol.36, No.11, pp.915-921, ISSN 0300-5712.

Forgie, AH. Pine, CM. Pitts, NB. (2002). The use of magnification in a preventive approach to caries detection. *Quintessence Int*, Vol.33, No.1, pp.13-16, ISSN 0033-6572.

Francescut, P. Zimmerli, B. Lussi, A. (2006). Influence of different storage methods on laser fluorescence values: A two-year study. *Caries Research*, Vol.40, No.3, pp.181-185, ISSN 0008-6568.

Guerrero, E. (2011). Validez y seguridad de las pruebas diagnósticas para la caries oculta de dentina: un estudio in vivo. Ph Thesis. University of Seville.

Hamilton, JC. (2005). Should a dental explorer be used to probe suspected carious lesions? Yes--an explorer is a time-tested tool for caries detection. *J Am Dent Assoc*, Vol.136, No.11, pp.1526-1530, ISSN 0002-8177.

Heinrich-Weltzien, R. Weerheijm, KL. Kühnisch, J. Oehme, T. Stösser, L. (2002). Clinical evaluation of visual, radiographic, and laser fluorescence methods for detection of occlusal caries. *Journal of Dentistry for Children*, Vol.69, No.2, pp.127-132, ISSN 0022-0353.

Heinrich-Weltzien, R. Kuhnisch, J. Oehme, T. Ziehe, A. Stosser, L. Garcia-Godoy, F. (2003). (Comparison of different DIAGNOdent cut-off limits for in vivo detection of occlusal caries. *Oper Dent*, Vol,28, No.6, pp. 672-680, ISSN 0361-7734.

Heinrich-Weltzien, R. Kuhnisch, J. Ifland, S. Tranaeus, S. Angmar-Mansson, B. Stosser, L. (2005). Detection of initial caries lesions on smooth surfaces by quantitative light-induced fluorescence and visual examination: an in vivo comparison. *Eur J Oral Sci*, Vol.113, No.6, pp.494-498, ISSN 0909-8836.

Hibst, R. Paulus, R. (1999). Caries detection by red excited fluorescence: investigations on fluorophores. *Caries Res*, Vol.33, pp.295, ISSN 0008-6568.

Hibst, R. Paulus, R. Lussi, A. (2001). Detection of occlusal caries by laser fluorescence: Basic and clinical investigations. *Medical Laser Application*, Vol.16, No.3, pp.205-213, ISSN 1615-1615.

Huysmans, MC. Longbottom, C. Pitts, N. (1998). Electrical methods in occlusal caries diagnosis: An in vitro comparison with visual inspection and bite-wing radiography. *Caries Res*, Vol.32, No.5, pp.324-329, ISSN 0008-6568.

Hyat, Tp. (1923). Prophylactic odontotomy : the cutting into the tooth for prevention of disease. *Dental cosmos*, Vol.65, pp.234-241, ISSN 0096-0187.

Kidd, EA. Ricketts, DN. Pitts, NB. (1993). Occlusal caries diagnosis: a changing challenge for clinicians and epidemiologists. *J Dent*, Vol.21, No.6, pp.323-331, ISSN 0300-5712.

Kidd, EA. Ricketts, DN. Beighton, D. (1996). Criteria for caries removal at the enamel-dentine junction: a clinical and microbiological study. *Br Dent J*, Vol.180, No.8, pp.287-291, ISNN 0007-0610.

Kuhnisch, J. Goddon I. Berger, S. Senkel, H. Bucher, K. Oehme, T. et al. (2009). Development, methodology and potential of the new Universal Visual Scoring System (UniViSS) for caries detection and diagnosis. *Int J Environ Res Public Health*, Vol.6, No.9, pp.2500-2509, ISNN 0960-3123.

Landis, JR. Koch, GG. (1977). The measurement of observer agreement for categorical data. *Biometrics*, Vol.33, No.1, pp.159-174, ISSN 0006-341X.

Llamas, R. Bonilla, V. Sánchez-Barriga, R. Pastor, C. Herrera, M. (2000). La caries, una enfermedad actual (II). Características morfológicas de la caries de esmalte no cavitada. *Rev Eur Odontoestomatol* , Vol.3, pp.129-40, ISSN 0214-8668.

Loesche, WJ. Svanberg, ML. Pape, HR. (1979). Intraoral transmission of Streptococcus mutans by a dental explorer. *J Dent Res*, Vol.58, No.8, pp.1765-1770, ISSN 0022-0345.

Lundberg, P. Morhed-Hultvall, ML. (2007). Twetman S. Mutans streptococci colonization and longitudinal caries detection with laser fluorescence in fissures of newly erupted 1st permanent molars. *Acta Odontol Scand*, Vol.65, No.4, pp.189-193, ISSN 0001-6357.

Lussi, A. (1991). Validity of diagnostic and treatment decisions of fissure caries. *Caries Res*, Vol.25, No.4, pp.296-303, ISSN 0008-6568.

Lussi A. (1993). Comparison of different methods for the diagnosis of fissure caries without cavitation. *Caries Res*, Vol.27, No.5, pp.409-416, ISSN 0008-6568.

Lussi, A. Imwinkelried, S. Pitts, NB. Longbottom, C. Reich, E. (1999). Performance and Reproducibility of a Laser Fluorescence System for Detection of Occlusal Caries in vitro. *Caries Research*, Vol.33, No.4, pp.261-266, ISSN 0008-6568.

Lussi, A. Megert, B. Longbottom, C. Reich, E. Francescut, P. (2001). Clinical performance of a laser fluorescence device for detection of occlusal caries lesions. *European Journal of Oral Sciences*, Vol.109, No.1, pp.14-19, ISSN 0909-8836.

Lussi, A. Megert, B. Longbottom, C. Reich, E. Francescut, P. (2001). Laser fluorescence may increase diagnostic sensitivity in detecting class I caries. *Journal of Evidence-Based Dental Practice*, Vol.1, No.2, pp.95-96, ISSN 1532-3382.

Lussi, A. Francescut, P. (2003). Performance of conventional and new methods for the detection of occlusal caries in deciduous teeth. *Caries Research*, Vol.37, No.1, pp.2-7, ISSN 0008-6568.

Lussi, A. Hellwig, E. (2006). Performance of a new laser fluorescence device for the detection of occlusal caries in vitro. *Journal of Dentistry*, Vol.34, No.7, pp.467-471, ISSN 0300-5712.

Matos, R. Novaes, TF. Braga, MM. Siqueira, WL. Duarte, DA. Mendes, FM. (2011). Clinical Performance of Two Fluorescence-Based Methods in Detecting Occlusal Caries Lesions in Primary Teeth *Caries Res*, Vol.45, pp.294-302, ISSN 0008-6568.

McComb, D. Tam, LE. (2001). Diagnosis of occlusal caries: Part I. Conventional methods. *Journal Canadian Dental Association*, Vol.67, No.8, pp.454-457, ISSN 0008-3372.

Mejare, I. Kallestal, C. Stenlund, H. Johansson, H. (1998). Caries development from 11 to 22 years of age: a prospective radiographic study. Prevalence and distribution. *Caries Res*, Vol.32, No.1, pp.10-16, ISSN 0008-6568.

Mejàre, I. Stenlund, H. Zelezny-Holmlund, C. (2004) Caries incidence and lesion progression from adolescence to young adulthood: A prospective 15-year cohort study in Sweden. *Caries Res*, Vol. 38, pp.130-41, ISSN 0008-6568.

Mendes, FM. de Oliveira, E. de Faria, DL. Nicolau, J. (2006). Ability of laser fluorescence device associated with fluorescent dyes in detecting and quantifying early smooth surface caries lesions. *J Biomed Op*, Vol.11, No.2, pp.024007, ISNN 1083-3668.

Ngaotheppitak, P. Darling, CL. Fried, D. (2005). Measurement of the severity of natural smooth surface (interproximal) caries lesions with polarization sensitive optical coherence tomography. *Lasers Surg Med*, Vol.37, No.1, pp.78-88, ISSN 0196-8092.

Nyvad, B. Machiulskiene, V. Baelum, V. (1999). Reliability of a new caries diagnostic system differentiating between active and inactive caries lesions. *Caries Res*, Vol.33, No.4, pp.252-260, ISSN 0008-6568.

Pastor, C. Lopez, G. Gomez, I. Sanchez-Barriga, R. Llamas, R. (1998). Valoración de los métodos de exploración de caries oclusales sin cavitación. *Rev Eur Odontoestomatol*, Vol.4, pp213-24, ISSN 0214-8668

Pereira, AC. Verdonschot, EH. Huysmans, MC. (2001). Caries detection methods: can they aid decision making for invasive sealant treatment? *Caries Res*, Vol.35, No.2, pp.83-89, ISSN 0008-6568.

Pitts, N. (2004). "ICDAS"--an international system for caries detection and assessment being developed to facilitate caries epidemiology, research and appropriate clinical management. *Community Dent Health*, Vol.21, 3, pp.193-198, ISSN 0265-539X.

Pitts, NB. Stamm, JW. (2004). International Consensus Workshop on Caries Clinical Trials (ICW-CCT)--final consensus statements: agreeing where the evidence leads. *J Dent Res*, Vol.83 Spec, No.C:C125-8, ISSN 0022-0345.

Pretty, IA. Maupome, G. (2004). A closer look at diagnosisi in clinical dental practice. Part 5. Emerging technologies for caries detection and diagnosis. *Journal Canadian Dental Association*, Vol.70, No.8, pp.540, ISSN 0709-8936.

Pretty, IA. (2006). Caries detection and diagnosis: novel technologies. *J Dent*, Vol.34, No.10, pp. 727-739, ISSN 0300-5712.

Reis, A. Mendes, FM. Angnes, V. Angnes, G. Grande, RH. Loguercio, AD. (2006). Performance of methods of occlusal caries detection in permanent teeth under clinical and laboratory conditions. *J Dent*, Vol.34, No.2, pp89-96, ISSN 0300-5712.

Ricketts, DN. Whaites, EJ. Kidd, EA. Brown, JE. Wilson, RF. (1997). An evaluation of the diagnostic yield from bitewing radiographs of small approximal and occlusal carious lesions in a low prevalence sample in vitro using different film types and speeds. *Br Dent J*, Vol.182, No.2, pp.51-58, ISSN 0007-0610.

Sheehy, EC. Brailsford, SR. Kidd, EAM. Beighton, D. Zoitopoulos, L. (2001). Comparison between Visual Examination and a Laser Fluorescence System for in vivo Diagnosis of Occlusal Caries. *Caries Research*, Vol.35, No.6, pp.421-426, ISSN 0008-6568.

Stookey, GK. Gonzalez-Cabezas, C. (2001). Emerging methods of caries diagnosis. *J Dent Educ*, Vol.65, No.10, pp.1001-1006, ISSN 0022-0337.

Thylstrup, A. Bruun, C. Holmen, L. (1994). In vivo caries models--mechanisms for caries initiation and arrestment. *Adv Dent Res*, Vol.8, No.2, pp.144-157, ISSN 0895-9374.

Toraman, M. Peker, I. Deniz, H. Bala, O. Altunkaynak, B. (2008). In vivo comparison of laser fluorescence measurements with conventional methods for occlusal caries detection. *Lasers Med Sci*, Vol.23, No.3, pp.307-312, ISNN 0268-8921.

Tranæus, S. Shi, X-. Angmar-Mansson, B. (2005). Caries risk assessment: Methods available to clinicians for caries detection. *Community Dentistry and Oral Epidemiology*, Vol.33, No.4, pp.265-273, ISSN 0301-5661.

Verdonschot, EH. van der Veen, MH. (2002), Lasers in dentistry 2. Diagnosis of dental caries with lasers. *Nederlands Tijdschrift voor Tandheelkunde*, Vol.109, No.4, pp.122-126, ISSN 0028-2200.

Weerheijm, KL. Gruythuysen, RJ. van Amerongen, WE. (1992). Prevalence of hidden caries. *ASDC J Dent Child*, Vol.59, No.6, pp.408-412, ISNN 0022-0353

Weerheijm, KL. Groen, HJ. Bast, AJ. Kieft, JA. Eijkman, MA. van Amerongen, WE. (1992). Clinically undetected occlusal dentine caries: a radiographic comparison. *Caries Res*, Vol.26, No.4, pp.305-309, ISSN 0008-6568.

Wenzel, A. Fejerskov, O. Kidd, E. Joyston-Bechal, S. Groeneveld, A. (1990). Depth of occlusal caries assessed clinically, by conventional film radiographs, and by digitized, processed radiographs. *Caries Res*, Vol.24, No.5, pp.327-333, ISSN 0008-6568.

Wenzel, A. Larsen, MJ. Fejerskov, O. (1991). Detection of occlusal caries without cavitation by visual inspection, film radiographs, xeroradiographs, and digitized radiographs. *Caries Res*, Vol.25, No.5, pp.365-371, ISSN 0008-6568.

Wenzel, A. Verdonschot, EH. Truin, GJ. Konig, KG. (1992). Accuracy of visual inspection, fiber-optic transillumination, and various radiographic image modalities for the detection of occlusal caries in extracted non-cavitated teeth. *J Dent Res*, Vol.71, No.12, pp.1934-1937, ISSN 0022-0345.

Wenzel, A. (1998). Digital radiography and caries diagnosis. *Dentomaxillofac Radiol*, Vol.27, No.1, pp.3-11, ISSN 0250-832X.

Wolwacz, VF. Chapper, A. Busato, AL. Barbosa, AN. (2004). Correlation between visual and radiographic examinations of non-cavitated occlusal caries lesions -- an in vivo study. *Braz Oral Res*, Vol.18, No.2, pp.145-149, ISSN 1806-8324.

Zandona, AF. Zero, DT. (2006). Diagnostic tools for early caries detection. *J Am Dent Assoc*, Vol.137, No.12, pp.1675-1684, ISSN 0002-8177.

7

Traditional and Novel Caries Detection Methods

Michele Baffi Diniz[1], Jonas de Almeida Rodrigues[2] and Adrian Lussi[3]
[1]Cruzeiro do Sul University,
[2]Federal University of Rio Grande do Sul,
[3]University of Bern,
[1,2]Brazil
[3]Switzerland

1. Introduction

Dental caries is a bacteria-associated progressive process of the hard tissues of the coronal and root surfaces of teeth. The net demineralization may begin soon after tooth eruption in caries susceptible children without being recognized by dental professionals. This process may progress further resulting in a caries lesion that is the sign and/or the symptom of the carious process. Caries is in other words a continuum which may by assessed falsely when only a certain time point is considered. Figure 1 shows different stages of the carious process.

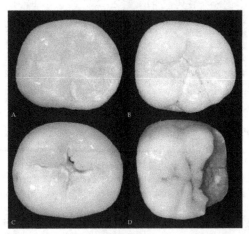

Fig. 1. (A) Sound occlusal surface. (B-D) Caries process in different stages.

Caries diagnosis implies more than just detecting lesions. Consequently, caries diagnosis - as an intellectual process - is the determination of the presence and extent of a caries lesion. Furthermore the judgement of its activity is an integral part of diagnosis.

Since diagnosis is a mental resting place on the way to treatment decision, it is intimately linked with the treatment plan to be followed. Thus diagnosis must include an assessment of activity because active lesions require active management (non-operative and operative treatment) whereas arrested lesions do not. The problem, however, is the assessment of the activity. The detection process may miss lesions (false negatives) or may overlook lesions that are present (false positives). The assessment of activity may be similarly wrong. For treatment decisions made in the clinic, the diagnosis should also express the individual patient's caries activity, which may be defined as the sum of new caries lesions and the enlargement of existing lesions during a given time (Wyne, 1993). It is a compound diagnosis comprising the immediate past caries experience, lesion progression and the clinical appearance of the lesions. The most important parameters for estimation of caries activity are the clinical appearance of a lesion and patient factors such as salivary flow, sugar intake and oral hygiene (Lagerlöf & Oliveby, 1996). Thus, caries activity can be evaluated by the assessment of factors associated with the pathogenesis of the disease and on the basis of data obtained from clinical examination. There are some clinical signs to get some idea of lesion's activity. An active initial lesion is dull and has a rough surface, it shows bleeding on probing in a patient with otherwise healthy periodontal conditions, it may be covered with plaque and on vestibular surfaces it is more adjacent to the gingival margin. An inactive lesion is shiny and has a smooth surface, and it is less adjacent to the gingival margin (Figure 2).

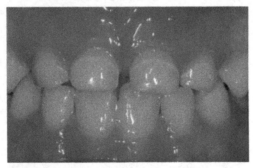

Fig. 2. Inactive carious lesion on the buccal surface. Note the shiny appearance and the position at some distance from the gingival margin.

Clinical-visual diagnosis may be amenable to longitudinal monitoring even though the assessment is qualitative. It would be easier to have a device that would not only detect demineralization but quantify it as well. Then monitoring progression or arrestment would be simple; use the device again and see in what direction the numbers change. The concept is hugely appealing so no wonder researchers have made such efforts to develop, test and perfect such devices. All these methods for caries detection are based on the interpretation of one or more physical signals. These are causally related to one or more features of a caries lesion. First, the signals must be received using a receptor device and classified. The classification of a signal is part of the diagnostic decision-making process. However, none of the methods is capable of processing all these signals to a status that could be called diagnosis. "The art of identifying a disease from its signs and symptoms" is a process that cannot be replaced by a machine or a device.

Caries measurement should be seen in the context of the objectives of modern clinical caries management and the continuum of disease states, ranging from sub-surface carious changes through to more advanced lesions (Figure 3). Measurement concepts can be applied to at least three levels: the tooth surface, the individual, or the group/population. According to Pitts (2004) modern clinical caries management can be seen as comprised by seven discrete but linked steps: (1) Caries detection represents a yes/no decision as to whether caries is present; (2) lesion measurement assesses defined stages of the caries process, taking into account the histopathological morphology and appearance of different sizes and types of lesion and the diagnostic threshold(s) being used; (3) lesion monitoring by repeated measures at a series of examinations is used when lesions are less advanced than the stage judged to require operative intervention of preventive care aiming either to arrest or to reverse the lesion to be assessed; (4) caries activity measures would be very valuable, but are relatively poorly developed and tested at present; (5) diagnosis, prognosis, and clinical decision-making are the important human processes in which all the information obtained from steps 1 to 4 is synthesized; (6) interventions/treatments, both preventive and operative, are now routinely used for caries management; and (7) outcome of caries control/management assesses caries management by examining evidence on the long-term outcomes.

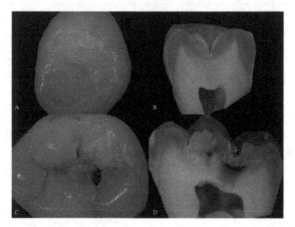

Fig. 3. (A) Initial carious lesion on occlusal surface. (B) Histological section through the lesion. The acid resistant and fluoride rich superficial layer is clearly visible. (C) Dentinal occlusal caries with cavitation and shadow. (D) Histological section through the lesion.

Early diagnosis of the caries lesion is important because the carious process can be modified by preventive treatment so that the lesion does not progress. If the caries disease can be diagnosed at an initial stage (e.g. white spot lesion) the balance can be tipped in favour of arrestment of the process by modifying diet, improving plaque control, and appropriate use of fluoride. Using non-invasive quantitative diagnostic methods it should be possible to detect lesions at an initial stage and subsequently monitor lesion changes over time during which preventive measures could be introduced.

2. Evaluation of the performance of caries detection methods

The performance of caries detection methods should be assessed considering two important parameters: reproducibility and validity. A reproducible method is the one that presents similar results and shows an agreement between two exams performed in different moments or by different examiners using the same sample. Reproducibility can be assessed by Cohen's Kappa test or Intraclass Correlation Coefficient (ICC).

Validity is the ability of a method of assessing what it is suppose to assess. It is calculated by the proportion of correct results taking into account the gold standard, which is the true and definitive diagnosis reference. Using these results, the validity of a method can be obtained by calculating values of specificity and sensitivity. Specificity is the proportion of cases classified by a method as negative (disease absent) considering the total of cases that did not developed the disease. Sensitivity, however, is the proportion of cases classified as positive (disease present) considering the total of cases that really developed the disease. The total percentage of correctly assessed cases considering the presence and the absence of disease is represented by the accuracy. Table 1 summarizes how sensitivity (Sn) and specificity (Sp) values can be calculated:

	Disease present (+)	Disease absent (-)	
Positive Test (+)	A	B	Total positive tests (A + B)
Negative Test (-)	C	D	Total negative tests (C + D)
	Sn%: A/(A + C)	Sp%: D/(B + D)	Total number (A + B + C + D)

Table 1. The generic 2 x 2 table used to calculate sensitivity (Sn) and specificity (Sp) values.

Concerning methods' validity and calculation of sensitivity and specificity values it is necessary to establish limits to define what "disease" and "healthy" mean considering the gold standard. These limits can also be called "cut-off points", which are combined according to the criteria used for the gold standard classification. For example, caries lesions can be classified in: (0) caries free, (1) caries extending up to halfway through the enamel, (2) caries extending into the inner half of enamel, (3) caries in dentin and (4) deep dentin caries. Therefore, cut-off points can be defined as follow:

D_1: all caries lesions are considered disease (1, 2, 3 and 4);
D_2: only caries lesions from the inner half of enamel are considered disease (2, 3 and 4);
D_3, D_4: only dentin caries lesions are considered disease (3 and 4).

3. Clinical and histological aspects of caries lesions on occlusal, approximal and smooth surfaces

The occlusal surface is characterized by the pit and fissure systems, a favorable biofilm stagnation area where the bacterial accumulations receive the best protection against functional/mechanical wear (mastication, attrition, abrasion from brushing, flossing or toothpicks). Those aspects contribute to the high prevalence of caries on occlusal surfaces both in the primary and permanent dentition (Kidd & Fejerskov, 2004).

The complex anatomy of the occlusal surfaces requires professional special attention and deep understanding of how lesions develop on this surface. It is known that the deepest part of the fissure usually harbors non-vital bacteria or calculus (Ekstrand & Bjørndal, 1997). An enamel caries lesion begins along the pits and fissures through acids diffusion from bacterial metabolism in the biofilm. This diffusion occurs through the side walls of the pits and fissures, guided by prisms direction and striae of Retzius. Histologically, the lesion forms in three dimensions and assumes the shape of a cone, with its base toward the enamel-dentin junction. Acids lead to the demineralization underneath the enamel surface and there is an enlargement in intercrystalline spaces, increasing its permeability. Over time, the surface porosity has increased and leads to a considerable increase of the lesion body (a subsurface lesion starts to form). Occlusal enamel breakdown is the result of further demineralization, thus leading to cavity formation (Nyvad et al., 2008).

The lesions on smooth surfaces result from an accumulation of biofilm along the gingival margins. Characteristically, those lesions follow the form of the gingival contour and can progress to form a cavity in enamel, and subsequently, that can extend through the dentin (Nyvad et al., 1999). In section, the smooth-surface lesion is conical as a result of systematic variations in dissolution along the enamel prisms. The conically shaped lesion represents a range of increasing stages of lesion progression, beginning with dissolution at the ultrastructural level at the edge of the lesion (Bjørndal & Thylstrup, 1995).

On the approximal surfaces, the biofilm accumulation occurs in the region below the contact point between the contact face and the gingival margin. The lesion may extend to the buccal and lingual directions, following the gengival contour (Nyvad et al., 1999). Histologically, the initial lesion in the approximal surface has a triangular shape with its base toward the outer surface and the apex facing the enamel-dentin junction. As mentioned earlier, this is because the acid diffusion from the bacterial metabolism is determined by the distribution of the biofilm and follows the direction of the enamel prisms (Nyvad et al., 2008).

Caries lesion on approximal surfaces in primary teeth presents a rapid rate of progression due to the morphologic characteristics of these teeth, making its detection difficult. Primary teeth have thinner enamel and dentin, lower mineralization rate, large dentinal tubules and larger contact proximal areas, which allow greater biofilm accumulation, and consequently, leading to initiation and progression of dental caries (Mortimer, 1970; Pitts & Rimmer, 1992).

4. Caries detection methods

The detection of carious lesions has been primarily a visual process, based principally on clinical-tactile inspection and radiographic examination. Caries detection methods should be capable of detecting lesions at an early stage, when progression can be arrested or reserved, avoiding premature tooth treatment by restorations. However, none of the conventional methods fulfill this requirement and are highly subjective. The development of some alternative non-invasive detection methods, such as laser fluorescence devices (DIAGNOdent and DIAGNOdent pen), quantitative light-induced fluorescence (QLF), fluorescence camera (VistaProof), LED technology (Midwest Caries I.D.), fiber-optic transillumination (FOTI), digital imaging fiber-optic transillumination (DIFOTI) and electrical caries monitor (ECM), can offer objectives assessments, where traditional methods could be supplemented by quantitative measurements.

4.1 Visual-tactile examination

Visual changes of the dental structure resulting from the demineralization process can be visually observed during caries development, such as an increase in opacity and roughness of the enamel.

Visual examination has been widely used in dental clinics for detecting carious lesions on all surfaces. This method is based on the use of a dental mirror, a sharp probe and a 3-in-1 syringe and requires good lighting and a clean/dry tooth surface (Hamilton, 2005). The examination is based primarily on subjective interpretation of surface characteristics, such as integrity, texture, translucency/opacity, location and color (Ekstrand et al., 1997; Nyvad et al., 1999). However, tactile examination of dental caries has been criticized because of the possibility of transferring cariogenic microorganisms from one site to another, leading to the fear of further spread of the disease in the same oral cavity. Moreover, use of an explorer can cause irreversible damages to the iatrogenic and demineralized tooth structure (Ekstrand et al., 1987; Stookey, 2005; Loesche et al., 1979).

Tooth separation can be used as a method for examination of a suspicious area on the approximal surface. With this technique an orthodontic elastic separator can be applied for 2-3 days around the contact areas of approximal surfaces, facilitating the clinical and probing assessments. However, this method might create some discomfort and requires an extra visit (Araújo et al., 1996). Studies have shown that tooth separation have detected more non-cavitated enamel lesions than visual-tactile examination without separation or bitewing examination (Hintze et al., 1998; Pitts & Rimmer, 1992).

Nyvad's system (Nyvad et al., 1999) is a reliable method for activity assessment of non-cavitated and cavitated caries lesions. According to this system, the examination is based only on clinical features of the surface (color, opacity and presence of discontinuities or cavitations), classifying the lesion as inactive or active. The original system used biofilm accumulation as an indicator for caries activity and used a sharp dental explorer to assess surface roughness. However, the Nyvad system was modified; adopting the use of a ball-ended probe should be gently drawn across the surface in order to assess its texture (rough or smooth) and also to remove the biofilm (Braga et al., 2009). If the lesion is active and cavitated, operative treatment is recommended. If active and non-cavitated, non-operative, preventive treatment is recommended (Nyvad, 2004). For detecting carious lesions, the examination should be mainly based on careful visual assessment on a clean/dry surface, without probing. An important aspect of caries detection is that the surface must be dry because saliva can mask differences in the reflection of light between carious and healthy tooth structure, hindering the observation of changes in color and brightness on the enamel surface. The criteria scores identify sound and active/inactive primary or secondary caries lesions. The Nyvad system has been shown to have good reproducibility and also construct and predictive validity for assessment of caries activity (Nyvad et al., 1999, 2003).

Visual examination has been show to have a high specificity but low sensitivity and reproducibility (Bader et al., 2001). Therefore, different criteria have been proposed to provide defined descriptors of different severity stages of caries lesions (Ekstrand et al., 1997; Ismail et al., 2007; Nyvad et al., 1999).

After the analysis of a systematic review presented in a conference in the USA and in the International Consensus Workshop on Caries Clinical Trials held in Scotland, it was concluded that the reliability and reproducibility of currently available caries detection / diagnostic systems, including visual and visual-tactile criteria, were not strong (Bader et al., 2001; Pitts & Stamm, 2002). Based on these findings, a new visual criterion has been introduced for caries detection.

The International Caries Detection & Assessment System (ICDAS) was developed and introduced by an international group of researchers (cariologists and epidemiologists) to provide clinicians, epidemiologists, and researchers with an evidence-based system for caries detection (Pitts, 2004). This method was devised based on the principle that the visual examination should be carried out on clean, plaque-free teeth, with carefully drying of the lesion / surface to identify early lesions. According to this system, the replacement of the traditional explorers and sharp probes with a ball-ended periodontal probe would avoid traumatic and iatrogenic defects on incipient lesions (Ekstrand et al., 2007; Ismail et al., 2007; Jablonski-Momeni et al., 2007).

ICDAS is a two-digit identification system. Initially, the status of the surface is described as unrestored, sealed, restored or crowned. After that, a second code is attributed to identify six stages of caries extension, varying from initial changes visible in enamel to frank cavitation in dentine (Ekstrand et al., 2007; Ismail et al., 2007; Zandoná & Zero, 2006). Some studies have shown good reproducibility and accuracy of ICDAS for occlusal caries detection at different stages of the disease in permanent (Diniz et al., 2009, 2011; Ekstrand et al., 2007; Jablonski-Momeni et al., 2007; Rodrigues et al., 2008) and in primary teeth (Braga et al., 2009; Neuhaus et al., 2010; Shoiab et al., 2009). The literature has suggested that the ICDAS criteria have potential to aid treatment planning (Diniz et al., 2011; Longbottom et al., 2009; Pitts & Richards, 2009).

ICDAS was developed with the mission to devise a set of international visual criteria for caries detection that would also allow assessment of caries activity (Ekstrand et al., 2007). The Lesion Activity Assessment (LAA) criteria have been developed for use in association with the ICDAS scoring system based on using weighted numerical values for lesion appearance (ICDAS score of the lesion), lesion location in relation to a cariogenic plaque stagnation area and surface integrity by tactile sensation when a ball-ended probe is gently drawn across the surface (Ekstrand et al., 2007; Varma et al., 2008). This evaluation involves the characterization of the caries lesion activity during a single clinical examination, in real time, in order to determine whether intervention is necessary (Ekstrand et al., 2009). The association of the LAA and the ICDAS codes involves lesion detection and coding, thereby estimating its depth or severity, and assessing its activity (Braga et al., 2009). An in vitro study found that there is no major difference between the Nyvad system and the ICDAS-LAA in assessing caries activity in primary teeth (Braga et al., 2009). However, in a clinical study ICDAS-LAA seems to overestimate the caries activity assessment of cavitated occlusal lesions in primary teeth compared to the Nyvad system (Braga et al., 2010).

Despite being the most widely used method in clinical practice, many studies have shown that visual-tactile examination should be associated with other caries detection methods, such as bitewing radiographs, especially for early caries lesions detection in approximal surfaces and for lesion depth evaluation on occlusal surfaces (Lussi, 1993; Lussi et al., 2006; Sanden et al., 2003; Wenzel, 2004).

4.2 X-ray based methods

The discovery of X-rays by Wilhelm Conrad Roentgen in 1895 provided a major advance in diagnostic imaging. In dental field, the North American dentist Edmund Kells began experimenting with radiography in 1986, becoming the pioneer of dental radiology.

Since then, the use of X-rays and radiographic films promoted a significant jump in the direction of dental therapy, since it provided substantial contribution in obtaining the diagnosis. In addition, radiographic techniques have been modified to acquire optimum X-ray quality and to increase diagnostic possibilities, as for detecting caries lesions.

4.2.1 Conventional radiography

Radiography is the most common caries lesion detection aid. It is fundamentally based on the fact that as the caries progress proceeds, the mineral content of enamel and dentin decreases, resulting in a decrease in the attenuation of the X-ray beam as it passes through the teeth. This feature is recorded on the image receptor as an increase in radiographic density. Clinically, the detection of carious lesions is based on a combination of visual-tactile and radiographic examination.

Bitewing radiography has been used for the detection and evaluation of caries lesions depth, which are invisible or poorly visible for inspection. Thus, radiography is mainly used for the detection of carious lesions in approximal surfaces, but is also recommended as a supplement for occlusal caries detection. However, experiments have shown that, once an occlusal carious lesion is clearly visible on radiographs, histological examination shows that demineralization has extended to or beyond the middle third of the dentin (Ricketts et al., 1995). Therefore, radiographic examination may underestimate the extent of caries lesions (Dove, 2001).

Bitewing radiography presents a tendency to make false-positive scores, and this could be due to the Mach-band effect, a perceptual phenomenon in which there is an enhancement of the contrast between a dark and a relatively lighter area, resulting in a dark band sharply demarcated (Berry, 1983). This effect causes an inclination to see radiolucency in the dentin-enamel junction where no dentin lesion is actually present (Espelid et al., 1994). Another effect, called cervical burnout, can be erroneously interpreted as cervical caries, once a collar or wedge-shaped radiolucency occurs between the bone height and the cemento-enamel junction (CEJ). This effect is an optical illusion phenomenon, due to the tissue density and the variable penetration of X-ray at the cervical region of the tooth and the regions above and below it, which produces a dark shadow on the radiograph due to lower absorption of photons in the neck of the tooth (Berry, 1983). For these reasons, radiographs should be interpreted with caution and requires constant retraining, updating, experience and information of the human observer (Diniz et al., 2010).

Several criteria are used to classify the extent of carious lesions on radiographs, such as (0) absence of radiolucency, (1) radiolucency in the outer half of the enamel, (2) radiolucency on the inner half of the enamel, which can extend up to the dentin-enamel junction (DEJ), (3) radiolucency in the outer half of the dentin and (4) radiolucency in the inner half of the dentin toward the pulp chamber (Mejàre & Kidd, 2008).

Regarding the performance of bitewing radiography, studies have found that the X-rays show a high sensitivity (50-70%) to detect caries lesions in dentin of both approximal and occlusal surfaces, compared to clinical visual detection. However, the validity of detecting enamel lesions is limited on the approximal surfaces and low for the occlusal surfaces (Wenzel, 1995, 2004). This difference can be explained by the fact that radiography is a 2-dimensional image of a 3-dimensional anatomy of the tooth structure. So, the superimposed cuspal tissues obscure initial changes in occlusal surfaces (Espelid et al., 1994; Neuhaus et al., 2009). In a systematic review of the literature, the evidence suggests that radiographs have high specificity and low sensitivity for caries detection. In other words, this means that there are great chances to occur false-negative diagnosis in the presence of caries than false-positive diagnosis in the absence of disease (Dove, 2001).

It is important to stress that many different factors can affect the ability of bitewing radiography to accurately detect lesions, such as technique, image processing, type of image receptor, exposure parameters, vertical and horizontal angulations of the X-ray beam, positioning of the film, display system, viewing conditions, possible distortions caused by the structures attached to the dental tissues and failures of interpretation, which can lead to an incorrect diagnosis (Dove, 2001).

Radiographic examination is useful in monitoring caries lesion development, in view of the fact that non-cavitated lesions can be reversed by non-invasive intervention, providing changes in mineral content of dental tissues. However, there are limits to the radiographic examination which should be considered, particularly since lesion behavior has changed, with cavitation occurring much later than previously (Pitts & Rimmer, 1992), Thus, it is worth remembering that radiography is not able to differentiate between an active and an arrested caries lesion, and to distinguish a cavitated and a non-cavitated lesion. According to Ratledge et al. (2001), 50-90% of dentin caries lesions radiographically observed on the approximal surface might present cavitation. There are cases where clinically "sound" and apparently intact occlusal surfaces, however, may develop lesions which penetrate into the dentin, sometimes named "hidden" caries (Ricketts et al., 1997), which can be observed only through radiographic examination (Figure 4).

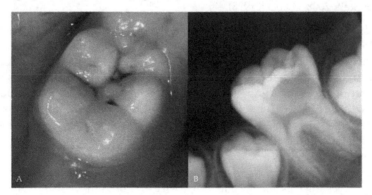

Fig. 4. Detection of occlusal caries. (A) Clinical aspect of a lesion in an intact surface. (B) Radiographic aspect of the lesion penetrating into the dentin – a typical "hidden caries".

Currently, there are some questions regarding specific indication of radiographs and intervals between subsequent radiographic examinations for caries detection. There is no evidence that routine radiographs will benefit a low caries risk population. In fact, this procedure can be harmful because it can induce a great risk of overdiagnosis, and consequently, an overtreatment. The frequency of taking radiographs depends on the individual caries risk, lesion activity and on the individual benefit to a patient (Neuhaus et al., 2009).

4.2.2 Digital radiography

Digital radiography is a complementary method that has been available in dentistry for more than 25 years, but digital imaging has not replaced conventional film-based radiography completely. Studies have shown that the number of dental professionals using digital radiography in clinical practice range from 11% to 30%. This fact can be attributed to the financial investment required to replace conventional radiography with digital imaging and also for the hesitancy to use a new technology, since it requires additional training on basic computer skills. On the other hand, a professional who is starting his/her career will not find huge differences in costs to acquire a conventional or a digital radiography system. Practitioners should remember that conventional radiography also involves costs for items, such as radiographic films, film mounts, processing solutions and time needed for cleaning the film processor (van der Stelt, 2008).

Studies have shown many advantages of digital radiography compared with conventional radiography. These include image acquisition process in real time, since the image is displayed immediately after exposure and no processing had to be performed. Other benefits include reductions in radiation dose (between 5% to 50% of the dose needed for conventional radiography) to obtain quality diagnostic images, time savings and digital manipulation of the image to enhance viewing, avoiding unnecessary or repeated radiographs. Digital images facilitate communication and case discussion among dental professionals, being a visual aid to be shown to the patient on the computer screen, increasing the confidence and credibility in the treatment-decision making process. However, the primary disadvantages of digital systems include the rigidity and thickness of the sensors, the high initial system cost and unknown sensor lifespan (Bin-Shuwaish et al., 2008; van der Stelt, 2008; Wenzel, 1998).

It is imperative to understand the digital radiography system to understand the principle of image manipulation. A digital image consists of a set of cells that are ordered in rows and columns, forming a table. Each cell is characterized by three numbers: the x-coordinate, the y-coordinate and the gray value. The gray value is a number that corresponds with the X-ray intensity at that location during the exposure of the digital sensor. Individual cells are called "picture elements", which had been shortened to "pixels". The numbers describing each pixel are stored in an image file in the computer. This feature is an essential difference between conventional and digital radiographs, once digital images can be modified after they have been produced. Thus, the user can apply mathematical operations (special algorithms or filters) to modify the pixel values, improving the image quality and modifying other characteristics, such as zoom, contrast, density and brightness of an image. The image numbers are converted into gray values and these are displayed on the computer screen as analog data. Then, the professional can assess and interpret the radiographic image produced (van der Stelt, 2008; Wenzel, 1998).

An example of useful image manipulation is the optimization of contrast and brightness of an image. This technique can be used to correct overexposure or underexposure of an image, although it is not an excuse to not pay attention to the correct exposure parameters. The manipulation can help to recover an image in which the exposure conditions were not optimal. This procedure may prevent the need for a radiograph remake, protecting the patient from an extra dose of radiation (van der Stelt, 2008).

Digital image presents lower spatial resolution when compared to the image obtained by conventional radiography. The extension or palette for digital images is normally limited to 256 shades of gray, while more than a million shades of gray may appear for conventional X-ray film. Therefore, it can be speculated that the performance of digital radiography for caries detection would not be superior to that of conventional radiography. However, the performance of digital radiography for caries detection can be improved with image manipulation possibility, such as contrast modification. Thus, digital radiography systems seem to be as accurate as the conventional radiography system. According to a literature review, digital radiography showed high sensitivity for detecting occlusal caries lesions into dentin (60-80%), with false-positives results of 5-10% (Wenzel, 1998).

Undoubtedly, as technology evolves, it is supposed that the performance of digital radiography will be improved in a near future. The development of different sensors and software will support the reliability and viability of digital radiography applications by dental professionals, bringing this method to daily practice.

4.2.3 Digital subtraction radiography

Digital subtraction radiography (DSR) is a more advanced image analysis tools. This method allows professionals to distinguish small differences between subsequent radiographs that otherwise would have remained unobserved because of overprojection of anatomical structures or differences in density that are too small to be recognized by the human eye. The procedure is based on the principle that two digital radiographic images obtained under different time intervals, with the same projection geometry, are spatially and densitometrically aligned using specific software. When the two images are registered and intensities of corresponding pixels are subtracted of the gray scale values, a uniform difference image is produced, resulting in a new image representing the differences between the two, called the subtraction image. In this new image, if there is a change in the radiographic attenuation between the baseline and follow-up examination, all the anatomical structures that do no change between radiographs are shown as neutral gray background, while regions that had mineral loss or gain are shown as a darker or brighter area, respectively (van der Stelt, 2008; Wenzel, 2004).

For a successful DSR, reproducible exposure geometry, and also identical contrast and density of the serial radiographs, are essential prerequisites. Long experience shows that this technique is very sensitive to any physical noise occurring between the radiographs and even minor changes leads to large errors in the results (Hekmatian et al., 2005).

Digital subtraction radiography has been used in the assessment of the progression, arrest, or regression of caries lesions. Subtraction consists of subtracting the pixel values of the baseline image from the pixel values of the second image. If the two digital images are identical, this method will produce an image without details (the result is zero). However, if caries has regressed or progressed in the mean time, the result will be different from zero. When there is caries regression, the outcome will be a value above zero (increase in pixel values). In case of caries regression, the result is opposite and the outcome will be a value below zero (decrease in pixel values) (Hekmatian et al., 2005).

Few studies are found in the literature investigating the DRS for caries detection. The system works well for approximal and occlusal lesions in dentin, indicating that this method presents high potential for dental caries research (Neuhaus et al., 2009).

Recently, a digital subtraction radiographic system was evaluated on occlusal surfaces (Ricketts et al., 2007). In this in vitro study, accuracy and reproducibility of DSR was compared to visual assessment of paired digital images in detecting changes in mineral content within occlusal cavities. Intra-examiner and inter-examiner reproducibility for detection of demineralization from the subtraction images was significantly better than viewing the paired images side by side. The subtraction radiography system used was found to be more accurate and reproducible than visual assessment of paired digital images, showing promising results for monitoring occlusal lesion progression in clinical studies.

It is important to clarify that DSR will not necessarily improve the detection of a caries lesion, but will only provide important information on any changes occurring over time, and is therefore, suitable for monitoring lesion behavior. As a new method, other studies should be carried out in order to validate its use in monitoring caries lesions.

4.3 Light-emitting devices

Other method used for caries detection is based on optical properties from sound and carious dental tissues.

Fluorescence is a phenomenon where the light is absorbed in a specific wavelength and then emitted in a higher wavelength. This characteristic has been observed in the dental tissues, since the pattern of light absorption and reemission (spectrum of fluorescence) of the dental tissues varies according to the excitation light wavelength (Benedict, 1928). Thus, light absorption and reemission is different in the enamel, dentin and cementum, as well as in sound and carious tissues. For this reason, fluorescence can be used for the detection and subsequent diagnosis of dental caries.

The natural fluorescence of hard dental tissues has been studied since long time ago. It is well known that as the enamel as the dentin shows an auto-fluorescence. In this way, caries lesions, dental plaque and microorganisms also show fluorescent components. It has been observed that the difference between natural fluorescence of sound and carious dental tissues can be quantified using light-emitting devices, such as laser, xenon or LED.

4.3.1 Laser fluorescence devices (DIAGNOdent and DIAGNOdent pen)

Laser fluorescence device is a non-invasive and quantitative method based on the laser-induced fluorescence. The first laser fluorescence device, DIAGNOdent 2095 (KaVo, Biberach, Germany), was developed in 1998 (Figure 5). It is based on the quantification of emitted fluorescence from organic components of dental tissues when excited by a 655nm laser diode (aluminum, gallium, indium and phosphorus - AlGaInP) located on the red range from the visible spectrum.

The emitted light reaches the dental tissues through a flexible tip. As the mature enamel is more transparent, this light passes through this tissue without being deflected. In contact with affected enamel, this light will be diffracted and dispersed. The later is able to excite either the hard dental tissue, resulting in the tissue autofluorescence, or fluorophores present in the caries lesions. These fluorophores derived from the products of the bacterial metabolism and has been identified as porphyrins (Hibst et al., 2001). The emitted fluorescence by the porphyrins is collected by nine concentric fibers and translated into numeric values, which can vary from 0 to 99. Two optical tips are available: tip A for occlusal surfaces, and tip B for smooth surfaces. This device has shown good results in the detection of occlusal caries, however, it might not be used as the only method for treatment decision-making process (Bader & Shugars, 2006; Rodrigues et al., 2008).

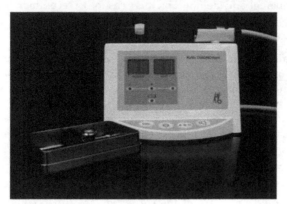

Fig. 5. DIAGNOdent 2095 – a laser fluorescence device for caries detection.

Recently, a new and compact device - DIAGNOdent 2190 or DIAGNOdent pen – (KaVo, Biberach, Germany) (Figure 6) has been introduced in the market. This device functions on the same principle as the earliest. For this reason, the device was condensed and the tips were modified. The tips used in this device are made from sapphire fiber and the same solid single sapphire fiber tip is used for propagation of the excitation and for collection of the fluorescence light, but in opposite directions and different wavelengths (Lussi & Hellwig, 2006). There are two tips which can be coupled on this device: an occlusal and an approximal tip. However, its performance in approximal surfaces is still limited. The device weights 140g and only one battery (1,5V) is needed.

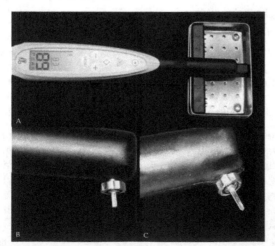

Fig. 6. (A) DIAGNOdent 2190 or DIAGNOdent pen calibration against the standard ceramic. (B) Occlusal tip. (C) Approximal tip.

As mentioned before, when a caries lesion or a dental surface is assessed by DIAGNOdent, a value between 0 and 99 is observed. This value is, theoretically, related to the lesion depth. For the values interpretation, several cut-off points have been proposed in the literature, as for DIAGNOdent as for DIAGNOdent pen. These cut-off points differ from each other in some units in the enamel and dentin. For this reason, is recommended that the clinician considers the values as an interval for the interpretation and also associates clinical and radiographic characteristics for the correct assessment of the lesions.

Other factor that might be addressed is the presence of stains due to inactive lesions or calculus on the occlusal surfaces due to biological sealing. Both can result in high values of fluorescence and, in consequence, false-positive results. Therefore, as also recommended before visual examination, cleansing of dental surfaces should be performed before laser fluorescence measurements. Besides, after professional prophylaxis using bicarbonate powder or prophylactic paste, it is important that the dental surface is rinsed off, so powder or paste does not remain in the fissure or inside microcavities. This could influence the laser fluorescence measurements (Diniz et al., 2011; Lussi & Reich, 2005).

In conclusion, the clinician who intends to use this method as a auxiliary in the caries detection process should be aware of the correct device functioning and remember that several factors might interfere the results, such as staining, calculus or powder/paste remnants; calibration procedures; and cut-off points variation for enamel and dentin caries.

For this reason, DIAGNOdent or DIAGNOdent pen should not be used as major method for caries detection, but as a supplementary tool for both visual and radiographic examination. Some situations, in which the professional is in doubt concerning the presence of a caries lesion on a surface free of staining, those devices can be suggested as substitutes for the radiographic examination. Besides, in the pediatric dentistry field, their use can also be suggested when X-ray examination is not possible due to the child behavior or during examination of patients with special needs or disabilities.

4.3.2 Quantitative light-induced fluorescence (QLF)

Quantitative light-induced fluorescence (QLF) (QLF-clin, Inspektor Research Systems BV, Amsterdam, Netherlands) (Figure 7) was developed for use in caries detection and it is available commercially for clinical use. This device consists of a handheld intraoral color microvideo CCD camera, interfaced with a personal computer and custom software (QLFpatient, Inspektor Research Systems BV, Amsterdam, Netherlands). The software enables to capture and to analyze in vivo images of the tooth during clinical examination.

QLF uses a 50-watt xenon arc-lamp and an optical filter in order to produce a blue light with a 290- to 450-nm wavelength, which is carried to the tooth through a light guide fitted with a dental mirror. The fluorescence images are filtered by a yellow high-pass filter ($\lambda \geq 540$ nm) and then captured by a color CCD camera (Al-Khateeb et al., 1997). When the tooth surface is illuminated by this high-intensity blue light, autofluorescence of the enamel is obtained by the intraoral camera, since all excitation light reflected or diffused is filtered. When a lesion is present on the surface, an increase in light scattering is observed relative to the surrounding enamel. The result of this is that the contrast between sound enamel and a carious lesion is improved with the lesion seen as being dark on a light green background (Neuhaus et al., 2009).

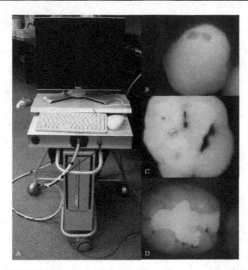

Fig. 7. (A) QLF system. (B) Fluorescence image of an enamel caries lesion on the buccal surface. (C) Fluorescence image of an occlusal caries lesion. (D) Fluorescence image of a secondary caries lesion around a composite restoration

To enable calculation of fluorescence loss in the caries lesion, the fluorescence of healthy tissue that was originally present at the lesion site is rebuilt by extrapolation of the fluorescence of healthy tissue that is found around the caries lesion. The difference between the lesion values and the reconstructed values allows the calculation of fluorescence loss. The fluorescence emitted is directly related to the mineral content of the enamel. Thus, the image can be used later to quantify the size, depth and volume of carious lesion produced by the parameters produced by the software: lesion area (in square millimeters), lesion depth - ΔF (percentage of fluorescence loss) and volume of carious lesion - ΔQ (the product of the lesion area in mm^2 and the lesion depth in percentage of fluorescence loss) (Zandoná & Zero, 2006).

Through these parameters, it is possible to detect and differentiate caries lesions at an early stage of development, making this system a sensitive method for quantification of enamel caries. Another advantage is that the image can be stored and used to motivate patients to seek healthcare and to prevent dental disease through education during routine preventive care. However, this method is more complicated, since the use of QLF consists of three main steps. The first is lesion detection by the examiner and subsequent capturing of an image of the lesion. Second, quantitative analysis is done of the image. Finally, the third step involves the long-term monitoring of the caries lesions, which enjoys the benefit of an innovative video repositioning part of the software, setting the initial image and the live image based on the geometry of similar fluorescence intensities. For that, it is necessary that the images of the tooth surfaces should be captured in the same position and angulation. Thus, same magnification images obtained at different observation times could be compared (Buchalla et al., 2001).

This fluorescence method has demonstrated that it can be reliably used by different examiners (Eggertsson et al., 1999). The literature demonstrates the diverse QLF applicability, such as detecting incipient primary lesions, secondary and root caries on smooth and occlusal surfaces in both primary and permanent teeth; detecting demineralization around orthodontic components; monitoring demineralization and remineralization caries lesion processes; quantifying dental plaque, erosion and fluorosis; monitoring caries removal; and detecting removal of extrinsic stains after tooth whitening (Al-Khateeb et al., 1997 ; Eggertsson et al., 1999; Neuhaus et al., 2009 ; Zandoná & Zero, 2006). However, it is important to emphasize that QLF can be influenced by some factors, such as stains, dental plaque, dental fluorosis or hypomineralization. Thus, as the presence of these confounding factors can produce images with similar appearance to that of dental demineralization, it is important that dental professionals should recognize those factors and differentiate them to perform a correct diagnosis.

QLF device has demonstrated potential to detect and longitudinally monitor caries lesions. In addition, it can provide dental professionals with significant information related to caries lesions severity. However, it should be emphasized that the information provided by QLF, as in all supplemental methods, can never be used by itself for clinical decision support. This information should be carefully evaluated and integrated to other individual patient factors and professional experience before making a definitive diagnosis and treatment plan.

4.3.3 Fluorescence camera (VistaProof)

Another device based on the light-induced fluorescence phenomenon is the intraoral camera VistaProof (Dürr Dental, Bietigheim-Bissingen, Germany) (Figure 8) that is based on six blue GaN-LEDs emitting a 405-nm light. With this camera it is possible to digitize the video signal from the dental surface during fluorescence emission using a CCD sensor (charge-coupled device). On these images, it is possible to see different areas of the dental surface that fluoresce in green (sound dental tissue) and in red (carious dental tissue) (Thoms, 2006). DBSWIN software is used to analyze the images and translate into values the intensity ratio of the red and green fluorescence. According to the manufacturer, those values are related to the lesion extension. The higher is the bacterial colonization, the higher is the red fluorescent signal. The software highlights the lesions and classifies them in a scale from 0 to 5, giving a treatment orientation in the first evaluation: monitoring, remineralization or invasive treatment. However, these values still need to be adjusted (Rodrigues et al., 2008, 2011). Recently, this device showed a good performance in detecting and quantifying dental plaque formed over smooth surfaces under high exposition to sucrose (Raggio et al., 2010).

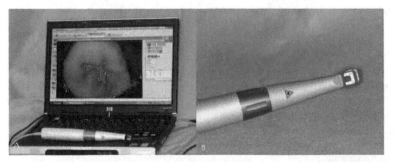

Fig. 8. (A) VistaProof fluorescence camera and DBSWIN software analysis. (B) Six blue LEDs emitting a 405-nm light.

An advantage of this method is that the patient can see in the computer screen the whole process of caries detection and visualize tooth areas where the disease shows more severe signals. This method makes easier the explanation to the patient concerning his/her clinical situation and possible available treatments. Besides, it is possible to monitor the caries lesion progression or arrestment overtime, as the images of the dental surfaces can be stored in the computer.

4.3.4 LED technology (Midwest Caries I.D.)

Recently, another device for caries detection was developed on LED technology - Midwest Caries I.D. - (DENTSPLY Professional, York, PA, USA) (Figure 9). The handheld device emits a soft light emitting diode (LED) between 635 nm and 880 nm and analyzes the reflectance and refraction of the emitted light from the tooth surface, which is captured by fiber optics and is converted to electrical signals for analysis. The microprocessor of the device contains a computer-based algorithm that identifies the different optical signature (changes in optical translucency and opacity) between healthy and demineralized tooth (Strassler and Sensi, 2008).

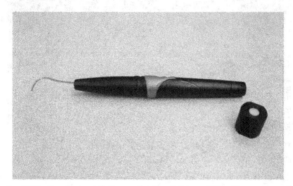

Fig. 9. Midwest Caries I.D. device and the standard for calibration procedure.

The demineralization leads to a change in the LED from green to red with a simultaneous audible signal, which is directly related to the severity of caries lesions. According to the manufacturer, when there is a change in the optical translucency and opacity of the dental tissues, the emitted green light changes to red and an audible signal could be heard. The faster the signal, the deeper the lesion. In the literature, there is only one published study which evaluated the Midwest Caries I.D. in vitro performance for occlusal caries detection (Rodrigues et al., 2011). In this study, the device presented the same cut-off limits for caries-free sites and enamel caries. This means that the Midwest Caries I.D. was not able to differentiate enamel lesions from sound surfaces.

4.3.5 Fiber-optic transillumination (FOTI) and digital imaging fiber-optic transillumination (DIFOTI)

Fiber-optic transillumination (FOTI) and digital imaging fiber-optic transillumination (DIFOTI) have been introduced to improve early detection of carious surfaces and have been accepted by clinicians as a supplementary tool during clinical examinations.

FOTI (Figure 10) device is a practical, easy, fast and inexpensive method of imaging teeth in the presence of multiple scattering. It is based on the changes in the scattering and absorption phenomenon of light photons that increases the contrast between sound and enamel caries. In other words, results from a local decrease of transillumination owing to the characteristics of the carious lesion. The illumination is delivered via fiber-optics from a light source to a tooth surface. The light propagates from the fiber illuminator across tooth tissue to non-illuminated surfaces. The resulting images of light distribution are then used for diagnosis. Its transmission can be observed either in the opposite side or in the occlusal surfaces, when molars and premolars are analyzed. As light scattering is higher in the demineralized enamel, it is possible to see the lesion as a dark area or a shadow. Besides, carious dentin appears orange, brown or grey underneath the enamel. This can help on the differentiation between enamel and dentin lesions. However, it has been show that FOTI diagnosis by naked eye can be subject to great inter- and intra-examiner variation (Neuhaus et al., 2009).

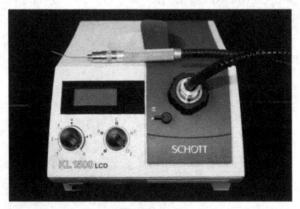

Fig. 10. Fiber-optic transillumination (FOTI).

To overcome the variability dilemma in FOTI, a new method has been tested. DIFOTI (Figure 11) is a method which employs digital image processing for quantitative diagnosis and prognosis in dentistry. It is based on light propagation just below the tooth surface and can be used to determine lesion depth. It uses fiber-optic transillumination of safe visible light to image the tooth. In this system, light delivered by a fiber-optic is collected on the other side of the tooth by a mirror system and recorded with a CCD imaging camera, instantaneously. Thus, DIFOTI images can be acquired in repeatable fashion by maintaining adjustment of a number of imaging control parameters. Then the acquired information is sent to a computer for analysis with dedicated algorithms, which produce digital images that can be viewed by the dentist and patient in real time or stored for later assessment. In addition, this system can use digital image processing methods to enhance contrast between sound and carious tissues and to quantify features of incipient, frank and secondary caries lesions on occlusal, approximal and smooth surfaces. It can also be used to detect other changes in coronal tooth anatomy, such as tooth fractures and fluorosis. DIFOTI presents higher sensitivity in detection early lesions when compared to the radiographic examination and has potential for quantitative monitoring of selected lesions over a period of time (Bin-Shuwaish et al., 2008; Young & Featherstone, 2005).

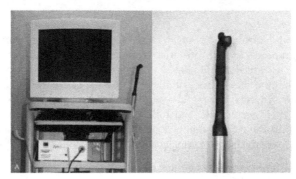

Fig. 11. (A) Digital imaging fiber-optic transillumination (DIFOTI). (B) Tip for occlusal surfaces.

4.3.6 Electrical caries monitor (ECM)

Over the last decades, the relationship between the extent of caries in teeth and electrical resistance has been investigated. It is possible to assess caries lesions considering the various parameters affecting the electrical measurements of teeth, such as porosity, surface area of the contact "electrode", the thickness of the enamel and dentin tissues, hydration of the enamel, temperature, ionic content of the dental tissue fluids, and the maturation time of the tooth in the oral environment (Neuhaus et al., 2009).

The studies on electrical caries monitor device (ECM) (Figure 12) have assessed these parameters in a "site-specific" or "surface specific" mode. This method has shown different results of reproducibility and validity (Huysmans et al., 2005; Kühnisch et al., 2006). Some in vitro studies indicated that the presence of stain is a confounder for ECM measurements. Besides, the different cut-off limits for enamel and dentin caries lesions may be needed for stained teeth (Côrtes et al., 2003; Ellwood & Côrtes, 2004). Therefore, its indication in the clinical practice is still uncertain. Further in vivo studies are necessary in order to make this technology useful in the practice.

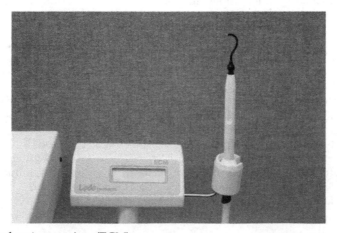

Fig. 12. Electrical caries monitor (ECM).

5. Conclusion

Visual examination, by observing clinical characteristics and appearance of the lesions, associated to radiographs is able to provide most of necessary information to the clinician for the detection of caries lesions. However, only severe and deep lesions are detected by radiographic examination. Therefore, auxiliary methods can contribute positively in the process of detection and their utilization should be encouraged. However, the clinician should be aware of their correct use and follow the manufacturer instructions. Besides, it should be kept in mind their disadvantages and affecting factors. This could provide more information for treatment decision-making process.

Moreover, it is important to state that the detection of caries lesions is only a part of the process of diagnosis. Other factors might be assessed, such as risk and caries activity, oral hygiene habits and fluoride exposition.

6. References

Al-Khateeb, S. ; Ten Cate, J.M, ; Angmar-Månsson, B. ; De Josselin de Jong, E. ; Sundström, G.; Exterkate, R.A. & Oliveby, A. (1997). Quantification of formation and remineralization of artificial enamel lesions with a new portable fluorescence device. *Advances in Dental Research*, Vol.11, No.4, (November), pp. 502-506, ISSN 0895-9374

Araújo, F.B.; Araújo, D.R.; Santos, C.K. & Souza, M.A. (1996). Diagnosis of approximal caries in primary teeth: radiographic versus clinical examination using tooth separation. *American Jounal of Dentistry*, Vol.9, No.2, (April), pp. 54-56, ISSN 0894-8275

Bader, J.D.; Shugars, D.A. & Bonito, A.J. (2001). Systematic reviews of selected dental caries diagnosis and management methods. *Journal of Dental Education*, Vol.65, No.10, (October), pp. 960-968, ISSN 0022-0337

Bader, J.D. & Shugars, D.A. (2006). The evidence supporting alternative management strategies for early occlusal caries and suspected occlusal dentinal caries. *Journal of Evidence-Based Dental Practice*, Vol.6, No.1, (March), pp. 91-100, ISSN 1532-3382

Benedict, H.C. (1928). A note on the fluorescence of teeth in ultra-violet rays. *Science*, Vol.67, No.1739, (April), pp. 442, ISSN 0036-8075

Berry, H.M.Jr. (1983). Cervical burnout and Mach band: two shadows of doubt in radiologic interpretation of carious lesions. *Journal of the American Dental Association*, Vol.106, No.5, (May), pp. 622–625, ISSN 0002-8177

Bin-Shuwaish, M.; Dennison, J.B.; Yaman, P. & Neiva, G. (2008). Estimation of clinical axial extension of class II caries lesions with ultraspeed and digital radiographs: an in-vivo study. *Operative Dentistry*, Vol.33, No.6, (November-December), pp. 613-621, ISSN 0361-7734

Bjørndal, L. & Thylstrup, A. (1995). A structural analysis of approximal enamel caries lesions and subjacent dentin reactions. *European Journal of Oral Sciences*, Vol.103, No.1, (February), pp. 25-31, ISSN 1600-0722

Braga, M.M.; Mendes, F.M.; Martignon, S.; Ricketts, D.N. & Ekstrand, K.R. (2009). In vitro comparison of Nyvad's system and ICDAS-II with Lesion Activity Assessment for evaluation of severity and activity of occlusal caries lesions in primary teeth. *Caries Research*, Vol.43, No.5, (September), pp. 405-412, ISSN 0008-6568

Braga, M.M.; Ekstrand, K.R.; Martignon, S.; Imparato, J.C.; Ricketts, D.N. & Mendes, F.M. (2010). Clinical performance of two visual scoring systems in detecting and assessing activity status of occlusal caries in primary teeth. *Caries Research,* Vol.44, No.3, (June), pp. 300-308, ISSN 0008-6568

Buchalla, W., De Josselin de Jong, E.; Ando, M.; Eggertssonn, H.; Lennon, A. & Stookey, G.K. (2001). Video-repositioning - increased repeatability for QLF caries monitoring method. *Journal of Dental Research,* Vol.80, No.1 Suppl, (March), pp. 115, ISSN 0022-0345

Côrtes, D.F.; Ellwood, R.P. & Ekstrand, K.R. (2003). An in vitro comparison of a combined FOTI/visual examination of occlusal caries with other caries diagnostic methods and the effect of stain on their diagnostic performance. *Caries Research,* Vol.37, No.1, (January-February), pp. 8-16, ISSN 0008-6568

Diniz, M.B., Rodrigues, J.A.; Hug, I.; Cordeiro, R.C. & Lussi, A. (2009) Reproducibility and accuracy of the ICDAS-II for occlusal caries detection. *Community Dentistry and Oral Epidemiology,* Vol.37, No.5, (October), pp. 399-404, ISSN 0301-5661

Diniz, M.B.; Rodrigues, J.A.; Neuhaus, K.W.; Cordeiro, R.C. & Lussi, A. (2010). Influence of examiner's clinical experience on the reproducibility and accuracy of radiographic examination in detecting occlusal caries. *Clinical Oral Investigations,* Vol.14, No.5, (October), pp. 515-523, ISSN 1432-6981

Diniz, M.B.; Lima, L.M.; Eckert, G.; Zandona, A.G.; Cordeiro, R.C. & Pinto, L.S. (2011). In vitro evaluation of ICDAS and radiographic examination of occlusal surfaces and their association with treatment decisions. *Operative Dentistry,* Vol.36, No.2, (March-April), pp. 133-142, ISSN 0361-7734

Diniz, M.B.; Sciasci, P.; Rodrigues, J.A.; Lussi, A. & Cordeiro, R.C. (2011). Influence of different professional prophylactic methods on fluorescence measurements for detection of occlusal caries. *Caries Research,* Vol.45, No.3, (May), pp. 264-268, ISSN 0008-6568

Dove, S.B. (2001). Radiographic diagnosis of dental caries. *Journal of Dental Education,* Vol.65, No.10, (October), pp. 985-990, ISSN 0022-0337

Eggertsson, H. ; Ferreira-Zandoná, A.G. ; Ando, M. ; González-Cabezas, C. ; Fontana, M. ; Martinez-Mier, E.A. ; Waskow-Chin, J.R.; Jackson, R.D.; Eckert, G.J.; Stookey, G.K. & Zero, D.T. (1999). Reproducibility of in vitro and clinical examinations with QLF (Quantitative Light-Induced Fluorescence). Developing guidelines for imaging and analyzing QLF images, and a process for training examiners. In: *Early detection of dental caries III: Proceedings of the 6th Annual Indiana Conference,* Stookey, G.K., pp. 213-228, Indiana University School of Dentistry, ISBN 0-9655 149-2-7, Indianapolis.

Ekstrand, K.; Qvist, V. & Thylstrup, A. (1987). Light microscope study of the effect of probing in occlusal surfaces. *Caries Research,* Vol.21, No.4, pp. 368-374, ISSN 0008-6568

Ekstrand, K.R. & Bjørndal, L. (1997). Structural analysis of plaque and caries in relation to the morphology of the groove-fossa system on erupting mandibular third molars. *Caries Research,* Vol.31, No.5, pp. 336-348, ISSN 0008-6568

Ekstrand, K.R.; Ricketts, D.N. & Kidd, E.A. (1997). Reproducibility and accuracy of three methods for assessment of demineralization depth on the occlusal surface: an in vitro examination. *Caries Research,* Vol.31, No.3, pp. 224-231, ISSN 0008-6568

Ekstrand, K.R.; Martignon, S.; Ricketts, D.J. & Qvist, V. (2007). Detection and activity assessment of primary coronal caries lesions: a methodologic study. *Operative Dentistry,* Vol.32, No.3, (May-June), pp. 225–235, ISSN 0361-7734

Ekstrand, K.R.; Zero, D.T.; Martignon, S. & Pitts, N.B. (2009). Lesion activity assessment. *Monographs of Oral Science,* Vol.21, (June), pp. 63-90, ISSN 0077-0892

Ellwood, R. &, Côrtes, D.F. (2004). In vitro assessment of methods of applying the electrical caries monitor for the detection of occlusal caries. *Caries Research,* Vol.38, No.1, (January-February), pp. 45-53, ISSN 0002-8177

Espelid, I.; Tveit, A.B. & Fjelltveit, A. (1994). Variations among dentists in radiographic detection of occlusal caries. *Caries Research*, Vol.28, No.3, pp. 169–175, ISSN 0008-6568

Hamilton, J.C. (2005). Should a dental explorer be used to probe suspected carious lesions? Yes – an explorer is a time-tested tool for caries detection. *Journal of the American Dental Association*, Vol.136, No.11, (November), pp. 1526, 1528, 1530, passim, ISSN 0002-8177

Hekmatian, E.; Sharif, S. & Khodaian, N. (2005). Literature review: digital subtraction radiography in dentistry. *Dental Research Journal*, Vol.2, No.2, pp. 1-8, ISSN 1735-3327

Hibst, R.; Paulus, R. & Lussi, A. (2001). A detection of occlusal caries by laser fluorescence: basic and clinical investigations. *Medical Laser Application*, Vol.16, No.3, (June), pp. 295-13, ISSN 1615-1615

Hintze, H.; Wenzel, A.; Danielsen, B. & Nyvad, B. (1998). Reliability of visual examination, fibre-optic transillumination, and bite-wing radiography, and reproducibility of direct visual examination following tooth separation for the identification of cavitated carious lesions in contacting approximal surfaces. *Caries Research*, Vol.32, No.3, pp. 204-209, ISSN 0002-8177

Huysmans, M.C.; Kühnisch, J. & ten Bosch, J.J. (2005). Reproducibility of electrical caries measurements: a technical problem? *Caries Research*, Vol.9, No.5, (September-October), pp. 403-410, ISSN 0002-8177

Ismail, A.I.; Sohn, W.; Tellez, M.; Amaya, A.; Sen, A.; Hasson, H. & Pitts, N.B. (2007). The International Caries Detection and Assessment System (ICDAS): an integrated system for measuring dental caries. *Community Dentistry and Oral Epidemiology*, Vol.35, No.3, (June), pp. 170-178, ISSN 0301-5661

Jablonski-Momeni, A.; Stachniss, V.; Ricketts, D.N.; Heinzel-Gutenbrunner, M. & Pieper, K. (2008). Reproducibility and accuracy of the ICDAS-II for detection of occlusal caries in vitro. *Caries Research*, Vol.42, No.2, (January), pp. 79–87, ISSN 0002-8177

Kidd, E.A. & Fejerskov, O. (2004). What constitutes dental caries ? Histophatology of carious enamel and dentin related to the action of cariogenic biofilms. *Journal of Dental Research*, Vol.83, No. Spec No C, pp. C35-C38, ISSN 0022-0345

Kühnisch, J.; Heinrich-Weltzien, R.; Tabatabaie, M.; Stösser, L. & Huysmans, M.C. (2006). An in vitro comparison between two methods of electrical resistance measurement for occlusal caries detection. *Caries Research*, Vol.40, No.2, pp. 104-111, ISSN 0002-8177

Lagerlöf, F. & Oliveby, A. (1996). Clinical implications: new strategies for caries treatment. In: *Early detection of dental caries: Proceedings of the 1st Annual Indiana Conference*, Stookey, G.K., pp. 297-321, Indiana University School of Dentistry, ISBN 0-9655 149-2-7, Indianapolis.

Loesche, W.J.; Svanberg, M.L. & Pape, H.R. (1979). Intra oral transmission of Streptococcus mutans by a dental explorer. *Journal of Dental Research*, Vol.58, No.8, (August), pp. 1765-1770, ISSN 0022-0345

Longbottom, C.; Ekstrand, K. & Zero, D. (2009). Traditional preventive treatment options. *Monographs in Oral Science*, Vol.21, (June), pp. 149-155, ISSN: 0077-0892

Lussi, A. (1993). Comparison of different methods for the diagnosis of fissure caries without cavitation. *Caries Research*, Vol.27, No.5, pp. 409-416, ISSN 0002-8177

Lussi, A. & Reich, E. (2005). The influence of toothpastes and prophylaxis pastes on fluorescence measurements for caries detection in vitro. *European Journal of Oral Sciences*, Vol.113, No.2, (April), pp. 141-144, ISSN 1600-0722

Lussi, A.; Hack, A.; Hug, I.; Heckenberger, H.; Megert, B. & Stich, H. (2006). Detection of approximal caries with a new laser fluorescence device. *Caries Research*, Vol.40, No.2, pp. 97-103, ISSN 0002-8177

Lussi, A. & Hellwig, E. (2006). Performance of a new laser fluorescence device for the detection of occlusal caries in vitro. *Journal of Dentistry*, Vol.34, No.7, (January), pp. 467-471, ISSN 0300-5712

Mejàre, I. & Kidd, E.A.M. (2008). Radiography for caries diagnosis. In: *Dental caries: the disease and its clinical management*, Fejerskov, O. & Kidd, E.A.M., pp. 69-89, Blackwell Munksgaard, ISBN 9781405138895, Oxford.

Mortimer, K.V. (1970). The relationship of deciduous enamel structure to dental disease. *Caries Research*, Vol.4, No.3, pp. 206-223, ISSN 0002-8177

Neuhaus, K.W.; Longbottom, C.; Ellwood, R. & Lussi, A. (2009). Novel lesion detection aids. *Monographs in Oral Science*, Vol.21, (June), pp. 52-62, ISSN: 0077-0892

Neuhaus, K.W.; Rodrigues, J.A.; Hug, I.; Stich, H. & Lussi, A. (2010). Performance of laser fluorescence devices, visual and radiographic examination for the detection of occlusal caries in primary molars. *Clinical Oral Investigations*, May 27 (Epub ahead of print).

Nyvad, B.; Machiulskiene, V. & Baelum, V. (1999). Reliability of a new caries diagnostic system differentiating between active and inactive caries lesions. *Caries Research*, Vol.33, No.4, (July-August), pp. 252–260, ISSN 0002-8177

Nyvad, B.; Machiulskiene, V. & Baelum, V. (2003). Construct and predictive validity of clinical caries diagnostic criteria assessing lesion activity. *Journal of Dental Research*, Vol.82, No.2, (February), pp. 117-22, ISSN 0022-0345

Nyvad, B. (2004). Diagnosis versus detection of caries. *Caries Research*, Vol.38, No.3, (May-June), pp. 192-198, ISSN 0002-8177

Nyvad, B.; Fejerskov, O. & Baelum, V. (2008). Visual-tactile caries diagnosis. In: *Dental caries: the disease and its clinical management*, Fejerskov, O. & Kidd, E.A.M., pp. 49-69, Blackwell Munksgaard, ISBN 9781405138895, Oxford.

Pitts, N.B. & Rimmer, P.A. (1992). An in vivo comparison of radiographic and directly assessed clinical caries status of posterior approximal surfaces in primary and permanent teeth. *Caries Research*, Vol.26, No.2, pp. 146-152, ISSN 0002-8177

Pitts, N. (2004). "ICDAS" -- an international system for caries detection and assessment being developed to facilitate caries epidemiology, research and appropriated clinical management. *Community Dental Health*, Vol.21, No.3, (September), pp. 193-198, ISSN 0256-539X

Pitts, N.B. (2004). Modern concepts of caries measurement. *Journal of Dental Research*, Vol.83, No. Spec No C, p. C43-C47, ISSN 0022-0345

Pitts, N.B. & Stamm, J.W. (2004). International Consensus Workshop on Caries Clinical Trials (ICW-CCT) -- final consensus statements: agreeing where the evidence leads. *Journal of Dental Research*, Vol.83, No. Spec No C, pp. C125–C128, ISSN 0022-0345

Pitts, N.B. & Richards, D. (2009). Personalized treatment planning. *Monographs in Oral Science*, Vol.21, (June), pp. 128-143, ISSN: 0077-0892

Raggio, D.P.; Braga, M.M.; Rodrigues, J.A.; Freitas, P.M.; Imparato, J.C. & Mendes, F.M. (2010). Reliability and discriminatory power of methods for dental plaque quantification. *Journal of Applied Oral Science*, Vol.18, No.2, (March-April), pp. 186-193, ISSN 1678-7757

Ratledge, D.K.; Kidd, E.A. & Beighton, D. (2001). A clinical and microbiological study of approximal carious lesions. Part 1: the relationship between cavitation, radiographic lesion depth, the site specific gingival index and the level of infection of the dentine. *Caries Research*, Vol.35, No.1, (January-February), pp. 3-7, ISSN 0002-8177

Ricketts, D.N.; Kidd, E.A.; Smith, B.G. & Wilson, R.F. (1995). Clinical and radio graphic diagnosis of occlusal caries: a study in vitro. *Journal of Oral Rehabilitation*, Vol.22, No.1, (January), pp. 15-20, ISSN 0305-182X

Ricketts, D.; Kidd, E.; Weerheijm, K. & de Soet, H. (1997). Hidden caries: what is it? Does it exist? Does it matter? *International Dental Journal*, Vol.47, No.5, (October), pp. 259-65, ISSN 1875-595X

Ricketts, D.N.; Ekstrand, K.R.; Martignon, S.; Ellwood, R.; Alatsaris, M. & Nugent, Z. (2007). Accuracy and reproducibility of conventional radiographic assessment and subtraction radiography in detecting demineralization in occlusal surfaces. *Caries Research*, Vol.41, No.2, pp. 121-128, ISSN 0002-8177

Rodrigues, J.A.; Hug, I.; Diniz, M.B. & Lussi, A. (2008). Performance of fluorescence methods, radiographic examination and ICDAS II on occlusal surfaces in vitro. *Caries Research*, Vol.42, No.4, (July), pp. 297-304, ISSN 0002-8177

Rodrigues, J.A.; Hug, I.; Neuhaus, K.W. & Lussi, A. (2011). Light-emitting diode and laser fluorescence-based devices in detecting occlusal caries. *Journal of Biomedical Optics*, Vol.16, No.10, pp. 107003-1-107003-5, ISSN 1083-3668

Sanden, E.; Koob, A.; Hassfeld, S. Staehle, H.J. & Eickholz, P. (2003). Reliability of digital radiography of interproximal dental caries. *American Journal of Dentistry*, Vol.16, No.3, (June), pp. 170-176, ISSN 0894-8275

Shoiab. L.; Deery, C.; Ricketts, D.N. & Nugent, Z.J. (2009). Validity and reproducibility of ICDAS II in primary teeth. *Caries Research*, Vol.43, No.6, (November), pp. 442-448, ISSN 0002-8177

Stookey, G. Should a dental explorer be used to probe suspected carious lesions? No – use of an explorer can lead to misdiagnosis and disrupt remineralization. *Journal of the American Dental Association*, Vol.136, No.11, (November), pp. 1527, 1529, 1531, ISSN 0002-8177

Strassler, H.E. & Sensi, L.G. (2008). Technology-enhanced caries detection and diagnosis. *Compendium of Continuing Education in Dentistry*, Vol.29, No.8, (October), pp. 464-465, 468, 470 passim, ISSN 1548-8578

Thoms, M. (2006). Detection of intraoral lesions using a fluorescence camera. *Proceedings of SPIE Lasers in Dentistry XII, Vol.6137*, No.5, pp. 1-7, ISSN 0002-8177

van der Stelt, P.F. (2008). Better imaging: the advantages of digital radiography. *Journal of the American Dental Association*, Vol.139, No. Suppl, (June), pp. 7S-13S, ISSN 0002-8177

Varma, S.; Banerjee, A. & Bartlett, D. (2008). An in vivo investigation of associations between saliva properties, caries prevalence and potential lesion activity in an adult UK population. *Journal of Dentistry*, Vol.36, No.4, (April), pp. 294-299, ISSN 0300-5712

Wenzel, A. (1995). Current trends in radiographic caries imaging. *Oral Surgery, Oral Medicine, Oral Pathology, Oral Radiology, and Endodontics*, Vol.80, No.5, (November), pp. 527-539, ISSN 1079-2104

Wenzel, A. (1998). Digital radiography and caries diagnosis. *Dentomaxillofacial Radiology*, Vol.27, No.1, (January), pp. 3-11, ISSN 0007-1285

Wenzel, A. (2004). Bitewing and digital bitewing radiography for detection of caries lesions. *Journal of Dental Research*, Vol.83, No. Spec No C, pp. C72-C75, ISSN 0022-0345

Wyne, A.H. & Guile, E.E. (1993). Caries activity indicators. A review. *Indian Journal of Dental Research*, Vol.4, No.2, (April-June), pp. 39-46, ISSN 0970-9290

Young, D.A. & Featherstone, J.D. (2005). Digital imaging fiber-optic trans-illumination, F-speed radiographic film and depth of approximal lesions. *Journal of the American Dental Association*, Vol.136, No.12(December), pp. 1682-1687, ISSN 0002-8177

Zandoná, A.F. & Zero, D.T. (2006). Diagnostic tools for early caries detection. *Journal of the American Dental Association*, Vol.137, No.12, (December), pp. 1675-1684; quiz 1730, ISSN 0002-8177

8

Clinical, Salivary and Bacterial Markers on the Orthodontic Treatment

Edith Lara-Carrillo

Faculty of Dentistry, Autonomous University of the State of Mexico,
Mexico

1. Introduction

Malocclusions are defined by different clinical signs, dental, aesthetic, functional and skeletal parameters. Numerous local factors can interfere with the adequate maxillary and mandible growth, which it can induce to the development of dentoskeletal alterations (Migale et al., 2009).

The Orthodontic or Orthopedic treatment is the indicated option to solve these problems; placement of fixed appliances in mouth increases risk of enamel demineralization; the braces, archwires, ligatures and other orthodontic appliances complicate the use of conventional oral-hygiene measures.

It is important to identify the changes in the oral environment in patients undergoing orthodontic treatment with fixed appliances, because in some cases involving long treatment duration and the clinicians are committed to preserving the oral health of the patient.

2. Particularities of the orthodontic treatment

Malocclusion is the third place in the oral diseases, the occurrence of occlusal anomalies varies between 11 al 93%; the complications that it brings could be: psychological derived from the alteration of the dentofacial aesthetics; oral function problems, including difficulties in the mobility of the jaw, pain or disorders in the temporomandibular joint and problems to chew, to swallow or to speak; and finally, problems of major susceptibility to traumatism, periodontal diseases or dental decay (Proffit, 2008; Sidlauskas & Lopatiené, 2009).

The orthodontic treatment can correct orofacial alterations, which can influence the patient's psique and social integration of the same one. Importantly, the face, the smiles and the teeth are part of the first impression of another person (Trulsson et al., 2002).

The purpose of the orthodontic treatment is to move the tooth as efficiently as be possible with the minimum of adverse effects to the tooth and the support tissues.

The requirements before initiating an orthodontic treatment are:

- Enough bone support (generally two thirds of the length of the root).
- To be sure that the occlusion will be stabilized at the ending of the treatment.
- The patient must have good health.

- The patient must be motivated and cooperator.

When placed fixed appliances, besides the brackets, the orthodontic technique use other attachments as: bands (actually preformed), wires, springs or buttons.

The length of orthodontic treatment with fixed appliances has approximately 13-15 months; nevertheless, factors so far linked to increased treatment duration include anatomy, malocclusion, direction growth, molar class, extractions, use of fixed appliances in both arches, and others (Turbill et al., 2001).

Patients who undergo orthodontic therapy have oral ecologic changes because increased retentive sites for retention of food particles, which allows the bacterial growth.

Lesions developed during orthodontic treatment could be radicular resorption, gingival recession and increase of caries risk and periodontal diseases. The enamel decalcification is one of the most common and undesirable complications of the orthodontic therapy. Some authors (Chang et al., 1999; Heintze, 1999; Zárate et al., 2004) show increase of decalcifications or white spot lesions in patient on treatment.

Demineralization of the enamel around brackets can be an extremely rapid process, which appears most frequently on the cervical and middle thirds of the buccal surfaces of the maxillary lateral incisors, mandible canines and the first premolars. The prevalence of new enamel lesions in orthodontic patients treated with fixed appliances and using fluoride toothpaste is reported to be 13 to 75 % (Derks et al., 2007).

We can find periodontal alterations after orthodontic treatment such as: generalized gingivitis after bonding and light lost of alveolar bone level and of epithelial insertion (Bollen et al., 2008).

It seems, that the bone lost could be more serious when more complex and extensive will be the orthodontic movement.

That is the reason because the maintenance of an effective oral hygiene is critical during the treatment.

We can considerate the next preventive measures in orthodontic patients:

- To evaluate the toothbrushing technique.
- To avoid the cariogenic diet.
- To evaluate the periodontal conditions during the treatment.
- To establish a continuos motivation for the oral care.

When we do a good orthodontic treatment and with a correct regime of oral hygiene, we do not have important periodontal complications.

It has been demonstrated that children who receive orthodontic therapy, at the end of this treatment, presents lower dental plaque levels and gingival bleeding that children who did not receive treatment; it could be because they have better dental alignment, but also to that the subjects modify his oral personal hygiene and attitude (Gwinnett & Ceen, 1979).

3. Caries risk markers on the orthodontic treatment

Diagnostic tests may serve multiple clinical objectives that benefit the individual patient. The clinician may use tests to: a) identify predisposing risk factors to modify risk and prevent disease; b) identify early disease-associated biochemical or physical changes prior to clinical signs of disease to halt the changes and reverse damage prior to loss of function; and c) determine which specific type of disease is involved to guide selection of the most effective therapy (Kornman, 2005; Sánchez & Sáenz, 2003).

Risk markers are biologic markers that either indicate disease or disease progression but are not causal or represent historical evidence of the disease, risk factors are characteristics of the person or environment that, when present, directly result in an increased likelihood that a person will get a disease and, when absent, directly result in a decreased likelihood of disease.

Risk factors for prediction of caries activity have been described by Featherstone (2000) and involve a balance between well-described pathological and protective factors. The pathological factors are primarily the levels of acidogenic bacteria, the frequency of fermentable carbohydrate ingestion, and the level of saliva flow. The protective factors include salivary proteins and antibacterial components, salivary composition of key minerals—for example, calcium and fluoride—and protective dietary components (Kornman, 2005; Featherstone, 2000).

About caries risk factors that it must be valued we can mention the following ones:

3.1 Clinical markers

To be able to evaluate the caries risk exist different markers, principally DMFT or DMFS index and bacterial counts (Streptococci mutans and Lactobacillus). The historical experience to caries that the patient presents by the DMFT or DMFS index is one of the most powerful predictor to caries risk. Nevertheless, it is well know that the caries is multifactorial and can change from a population to other one, from an individual to other one even from a group of teeth to other one.

3.1.1 DMFS index

The DMFT index was developed by Klein, Palmer and Knutson during a study of the dental condition and the need of children's treatment in elementary schools in Hagerstown, Maryland, USA, in 1935. It has been the most important index in the dental researches to quantify the prevalence of tooth decay (Katz et.al., 1997).

The caries experience (past and present) indicates the teeth damages and treatments received before by the count of teeth decays or natural history of the dental caries, which it expresses as decayed, missing and filled teeth (DMFT index) or decayed, missing and filled surfaces (DMFS index), both indexes express numerically the caries prevalence. The sum of these three points is the index (Sánchez & Sáenz, 1998; World Health Organization [WHO], 1997; WHO, 2011b).

For better analysis and interpretation it will be separate in each component and express it by percentage or mean. This is important to compare populations.

To obtain DMFT index in population, WHO recommended the next age groups: 5-6, 12, 15, 18, 35-44, 60-74 years. The index at 12 age is used to compare the oral health between countries.

The scientific evidences suggest that this is the most sensitive indicator to predict future risk, since if a subject does not establish the biochemical balance between demineralization-remineralization it will develop more caries lesions.

World Health Organization clearly established the methodology to obtain the index in the Oral Health Surveys. As increase the lesions number, increases the risk to develop caries, even in filled teeth (WHO, 1997).

The subjects are examined in the clinic area with the aid of a dental mouth mirror and periodontal probe, type E. The presence of caries was recorded using WHO's DMFS criteria.

For permanent dentition use the next codes:

Codes	Condicion
0	Health
1	Decayed
2	Filled with caries
3	Filled without caries
4	Missing by caries
5	Missing by other reason
6	Sealant, coat
7	Bridge or crown
8	Non eruption
9	Exclude

0: showing no evidence of either treated or untreated caries. A crown may have defects and still be recorded as 0. Defects that can be disregarded include white spots; discolored or rough spots that are not soft; stained enamel pits or fissures; dark, shiny, hard, pitted areas of moderate to severe fluorosis; or abraded areas.

1: indicates a tooth with caries. A tooth or root with a definite cavity, undermined enamel, or detectably softened or leathery area of enamel or cementum can be designated a 1. A tooth with a temporary filling, and teeth that are sealed but decayed, are also termed 1.

2: Filled teeth, with additional decay. No distinction is made between primary caries which is not associated with a previous filling, and secondary caries, adjacent to an existing restoration.

3: indicates a filled tooth with no decay. If a tooth has been crowned because of previous decay, that tooth is judged a 3. When a tooth has been crowned for another reason such as aesthetics or for use as a bridge abutment, a 7 is used.

4: indicates a tooth that is missing as a result of caries. When primary teeth are missing, the score should be used only if the tooth is missing prematurely. Primary teeth missing because of normal exfoliation need no recording.

5: a permanent tooth missing for any other reason than decay is given a 5. Examples are teeth extracted for orthodontics or periodontal disease, teeth that are congenitally missing, or teeth missing by trauma.

6: is assigned to teeth on which sealants have been placed. Teeth on which the occlusal fissure has been enlarged and a composite material placed should also be termed 6.

7: is used to indicate that the tooth is part of a fixed bridge. When a tooth has been crowned for a reason other than decay, this code is also used. Teeth that have veneers or laminates covering the facial surface are also termed 7 when there is no evidence of caries or restoration. A 7 is also used to indicate a root replaced by an implant. Teeth that have been replaced by bridge pontics are scored 4 or 5; their roots are scored 9.

8: this code is used for a space with an unerupted permanent tooth where no primary tooth is present. The category does not include missing teeth.

9: Erupted teeth that cannot be examined — because of orthodontic bands, for example — are scored a 9.

The "D" of DMFT refers to all teeth with codes 1 and 2. The "M" applies to teeth scored 4 in subjects under age 30, and teeth scored 4 or 5 in subjects over age 30. The "F" refers to teeth with code 3. Those teeth coded 6, 7, 8, 9, or T are not included in DMFT calculations.

The parameters to reference are:

Low   1 to 3 caries lesions
Moderate   4 to 6 caries lesions
High   7 to 9 caries lesions
Higher   10 or mores caries lesions (Fig. 1).

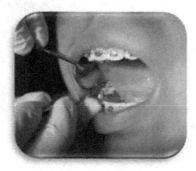

Fig. 1. Obtained DMFS index.

3.1.2 Supragingival plaque

The dental plaque represents a bacterial structure formed in the surfaces of the teeth that cannot be eliminated by water, which contains great number of microorganisms grouped and surrounded with extracellular materials from bacterial and salivary origin.

It has two phases related between them: inner one, with the enamel, where they find salivary free components of cells forming a cuticle or cap named biofilm and another in contact with the oral cavity, named interface plaque - saliva. If a tooth is cleaned deeply, exposing the enamel to the oral environment, in less than one hour this one would remain covered by the biofilm, whereas the initial formation of the dental plaque can need up to two hours. (Harris & García-Godoy, 2001; Menaker et al., 1986)

The principal diseases originated by dental plaque are caries and periodontal diseases, they originate in sites where the dental plaque is more abundant and is stagnant.

A number of plaque indices have been developed for assessing individual levels of plaque control and are also have been used in several epidemiological studies. Some of the most well - known indices, which have been used in numerous studies, are listed below:

- Oral Hygiene Index (Greene and Vermillion, 1960)
- Simplified Oral Hygiene Index (OHI-S, Greene and Vermillion, 1964)
- Silness-Löe Index (Silness and Löe, 1964)
- Quigley Hein Index (Modified by Turesky et al, 1970)
- The Plaque Control Record (O' Leary T, Drake R, Naylor, 1972).

The plaque control record evaluating the presence of soft debris on the tooth surfaces and dentogingival junction, as well as toothbrushing efficacy. (Butler et al., 1996; O'Leary et al., 1972).

According to O'Leary index, plaque is disclosed with a chewable tablet and its amount estimated. To determine an individual's score, the clinician multiplies the number of surfaces with plaque by 100, and divides that by the number of tooth surfaces examined. (WHO, 2011a) (Fig. 2).

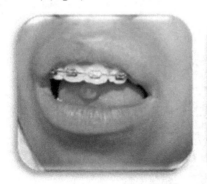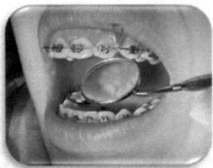

Fig. 2. Plaque control record.

3.2 Salivary markers

Saliva is a fluid present in mouth that comes from major and minor glands. Saliva is essential for the protection of the tooth against dental caries and protects the integrity of the soft oral tissues, facilitates the mastication, the swallowing and the speech, as well as the sensibility and the digestive functions in the oral cavity. Near 99 % of saliva is water, 1% remaining consists of a complex mixture of constituent to different concentrations (Harris & García Godoy, 2001; Featherstone, 2000; Fenoll-Palomares et al., 2004; Larmas, 1992; Leone, 2001).

The principal functions of the saliva are:

1. Protection functions (lubrication, preserve the integrity of the oral mucous, cleanliness, buffer capacity, dental remineralization and antimicrobial).

2.   Functions related to the mastication and the speech (food preparation by the digestion, flavor and phonation) (Kaufman & Lamster, 2000).

To evaluate the quantity of production as well as his functions helps us to determine factors of the guest in the development of dental decay.

3.2.1 Unstimulated saliva

The average of total saliva flow is 0.3 to 0.4 ml/min in adults, exist approximately a saliva secretion of 1500 ml/24 hrs. This rate of unstimulated saliva flow is based to a circadian rhythm, with a major flow in the middle of the evening and minor about 4 a.m. The flow changes considerably in persons who are resting. During sleep, the flow is very low or non-existent and increases during the day, especially with the food ingestion.

An unstimulated salivary <0.30 mL/min it is considered like risk factor (Ansai et al., 1994; Harris & García-Godoy, 2001; Fenoll-Palomares et al., 2004; Larmas, 1992; Leone, 2001; Zárate et al., 2004).

All salivary components neutralize the acids produced by cariogenic bacterias. For this reason the saliva production is important to support the oral health. Any agent or condition that reduces the quantity of saliva increases the risk of dental decay.

One way to measure this is by the formation time (in seconds) of small saliva drops in the inner mucous of the lower lip and compared with a chart. (Saliva Check®[1]) (Varma et al., 2008) (Fig. 3)

Low   greater than 60 seconds
Normal   30 a 60 seconds
High   less than30 seconds

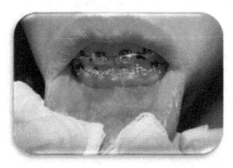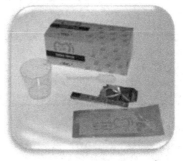

Fig. 3. Unstimulated saliva flow measured by Kit Saliva Check.

3.2.2 Stimulated saliva

Physiologically the stimulus can be mechanic as mastication. It can be gustatory as result of the stimulation of the gustatory or psychological papilla on having imagined the favorite food. Inversely, it can diminish with fear, radiation causing destruction of the salivary

---

[1] Saliva Check®, GC America Inc., Alsip, IL, USA.

glands, thyroid insufficiency, Sjögren's syndrome or medicaments (neuroleptics, antidepressants and antihypertensives) (Harris & García-Godoy, 2001) (Fig. 4)

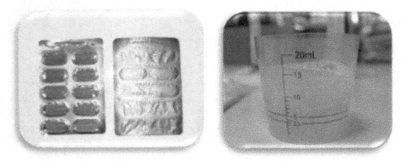

Fig. 4. Stimulated salivary flow.

Stimulated saliva could be obtained during 5 minutes by chewing an unflavored piece of wax or chewing gum; the result was expressed in mL/min. With a moderate stimulation, it can collect 1 to 2 mL/min. When the stimulated salivary flow is lower than 0.7 ml/min, it could be xerostomia with a caries risk (Harris & García-Godoy, 2001; Heintze et al., 1999).

3.2.3 Salivary pH

Salivary pH is the acidity or alcalinity of the saliva, normally presents a pH of 6.3, but could be modified by the oral health (Prieto & Yuste, 2010).

If salivary pH diminished can increase the enamel demineralization. There is no exist an exact pH at which demineralization begins, it may be in the range of 5.5 to 5.0 (critical pH). This is a very large range due to the mineralization is given according to pH and duration of exposure of the enamel surface to the acid environment (Anderson et al., 2001; Dawes, 2003).

The concept of critical pH is applicable only to solutions that are in contact with a particular mineral, such as enamel. Saliva and plaque fluid, for instance, are normally supersaturated with respect to tooth enamel because the pH is higher tan the critical pH, so our teeth do not dissolve in our saliva or under plaque (Featherstone, 2000; Dawes, 2003) (Fig. 5).

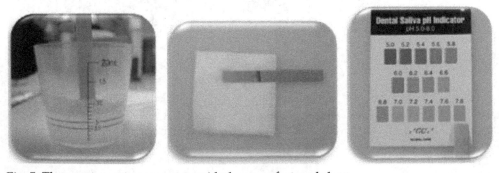

Fig. 5. The reactive strip comparate with the manufactured chart.

To determine salivary pH, you can use a ph-meter or by the reactive strip.

The Saliva Check®1 reactive strip is submerged in stimulated saliva for 10 to 20 seconds and the color obtained is compared with categorical levels in the chart:

Highly acidic   red section (pH de 5.0 to 5.8)
Moderately acidic   yellow section (pH de 6.0 to 6.6)
Healthy saliva   green section (pH de 6.8 to 7.8).

3.2.4 Buffer capacity

Buffer capacity is the saliva ability to neutralize acids, salivary pH back to normal parameters after bacterial acidogenesis. After exposure to fermentable carbohydrate occur a series of reactions with decreasing pH, as it decreases, some salivary minerals and proteins are liberate to avoid the salivary pH drop. Increased salivary buffering minimizes the final products of the acidogenic bacteria. Magnesium and carbonate ions are adsorbed to the enamel crystals, and then they are dissolved and added to the oral environment. Even calcium and phosphate ions are available for remineralization when the pH begins to return to normal parameters.

If acid production continues after 30 to 45 minutes, the pH rises and minerals in ionic form incorporate into the tooth structure. At this time reverse the demineralization process (Monterde et al., 2001).

This salivary function is one of the best indicators of caries susceptibility because it reveals the host response. Patients with high buffering capacity are resistant to the caries process. The low capacity may indicate: decreased salivary flow, reduced host response to cariogenic agents, possible malnutrition or pregnancy (Larmas, 1992).

Buffer capacity might be determined quickly placing stimulated saliva using a pipette in the reactive strip of the Saliva Check®1 test and will be compared with the chart after 2 minutes; the final result was obtained by adding the scores of 3 reactive zones:

Green   4 points
Green/blue   3 points
Blue   2 points
Red/blue   1 point
Red   0 points (Fig. 6).

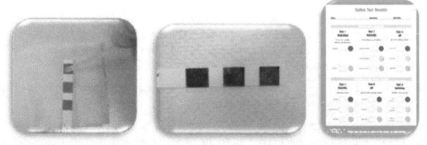

Fig. 6. Buffering capacity (Saliva Check®).

Interpreting the result:

Very low	0 to 5 points
Low	6 to 9 points
Normal/High	10 to 12 points

3.3 Bacterial markers

The acids produced by bacterial fermentation in plaque dissolve the mineral matrix of the tooth. A reversible chalk-white spot is the first manifestation of the carious lesion, which can lead to cavitation if the mineral continues to be exposed to acid. Early detection of carious lesions provides a great opportunity to limit enamel demineralization associated with this process.

3.3.1 Streptococus mutans

Streptococcus mutans are bacterias that grow in chains or in pairs, no movement, non-spore forming and usually react positively to Gram test. The name given by the tendency to change shape, can be found as spheres or more elongated, like bacillus.

There are numerous reports of a positive correlation between the presence of mutans streptococci and caries increase (Ansai et al., 1994; Heintze et al., 1999; Larmas, 1992; Niwa & Fukuda, 1989; Tanzer et al., 2001).

Streptococcus mutans are the most important bacterias at the beginning of the caries, colonize the host only after the first tooth erupts, are acquired primarily by direct transmission from mothers, have a preference for the occlusal surfaces of molars and interproximal areas of teeth and lack of ability to adhere to the oral soft tissues (National Institutes of Health Consensus, 2001).

The action of Streptococcus mutans, occurs in three phases: 1) initial interaction with the tooth surface via adhesins, 2) the colonization and growth of cariogenic bacteria in the film and 3) the production of glucose and glucans by the bacterial enzyme glucosyltransferase, which is involved into formation of lactic acid and initiates the process of demineralization of the tooth (Anusavice, 2005).

Microorganisms are more involved in the formation of cavities by their own virulence factors: acidogenicity, aciduric (acid produced in a medium with low pH) and acidophilus (resists the acidity of the medium).

Diverse tests based predominantly on quantitative estimation of Streptococcus mutans per milliliter of saliva (colony-forming unit [CFU]/mL): MSBB method (Matsukubo et al.), Caries Screen SM (Jordan et al.) and Dentocult® SM (Orion Diagnostica, Espoo, Finland) according to Jensen and Bratthall (1989).

These three are based on the fact that bacitracin inhibits the growth of other oral streptococci except mutans on mitis salivarius medium (Fig. 7).

A recently developed Streptococcus mutans detection system, Saliva-Check SM® (GC America, USA), eliminates the need for an incubation period. It can detect salivary S. mutans levels in 30 minutes.

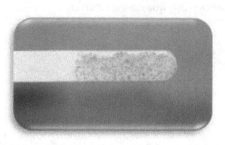
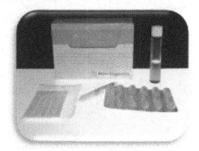

Fig. 7. Dentocult SM® strip mutans.

The average value for any possibility of decay should be more than 250,000 colony-forming unit (CFU) per milliliter of saliva, the higher values of 1'000, 000 CFU / mL indicate a high risk of caries (Heintze et al., 1999).

The bacitracin disc may be placed in the selective culture Dentocult® SM[2]; 15 minutes before sampling. Let the patient chew a paraffin pellet for 1 minute. This stimulates the secretion of saliva and transfers mutans streptococci from toothsurfaces into the saliva. Press the rough surface of the strip against the saliva remaining on the patient's tongue (Fig. 8).

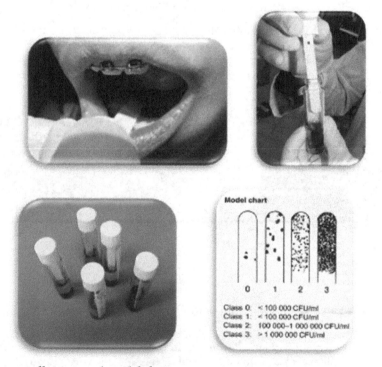

Fig. 8. Specimen collection, and model chart.

---

[2] Dentocult® SM Strip Mutans (Orion Diagnostica, Helsinki, Finland)

Incubate the vial at 37° C for 48 hours with the cap one quarter of a turn open. Interpretation of results according following score:

0   negative or < 100 000 CFU/mL,
1   100 000 to 1 000 000 CFU/mL,
2   10^5 to 10^6 CFU/mL,
3   >1 000 000 CFU/mL

3.3.2 Lactobacillus

Lactobacillus is considered secondary invaders, can contribute to tooth demineralization once they are established carious lesions. Lactobacilli can be found in the mouth before the teeth erupt, even when the diet is rich in fermentable carbohydrates and no active carious lesions.

They are present in small numbers on the plaque and tend to be found in saliva and in deep carious lesions. Weakly bind to the enamel surfaces, are lazy in their nutritional requirements, are acidogenic and aciduric. They are located in the undercut areas of the tooth, such as defects or margins of fillings or orthodontic bands (Ansai et al., 1994; Heintze et al., 1999; Menaker et al., 1986; Tanzer et al., 2001).

The development of caries should be considered in two-stage process: in Streptococcus mutans involved in lesion initiation and lactobacilli in progression it.

The standard method for determining the presence of lactobacilli is through the selective medium Rogosa SL agar. An alternative was established by Larmas in 1975 with the introduction of the test Dentocult LB®. The advantage is that it can be used in the dental office and the results can be shown to make the patient aware of the presence of lactobacilli in the mouth (Fig. 9).

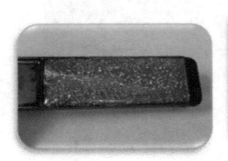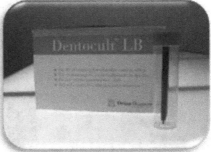

Fig. 9. Dentocult LB® test.

Values greater than 100,000 CFU / mL indicate a high risk of caries (Heintze et al., 1999; Larmas, 1992).

Dentocult® LB[3] procedure (Fig. 10) consists in pour the collected saliva over both agar surfaces, ensuring that they are well moistened. If the saliva is very viscous, the sample can also be applied using a sterile swab, then screw the slide tightly back into the tube and place

---

[3] Dentocult® LB (Orion Diagnostica, Helsinki, Finland)

the tube in an incubator for 72 hours at 37° C. To obtain a colony count remove the slide from the tube and compare the colony density with the model chart provided in the kit:

NC   Non count or few colonies
0   1 000 UFC/ml (low)
1   10 000 UFC/ml (medium)
2   100 000 UFC/ml (high)
3   1 000 000 UFC/ml (higher)

Actually exists the CRT bacteria test (Ivoclar Vivadent AG, Schaan, Liechtenstein) which allows clearly identify and semi-quantitatively determine both cariogenic bacterias.

Prognosis of caries becomes more effective when the lactobacilli and streptococci tests are combined.

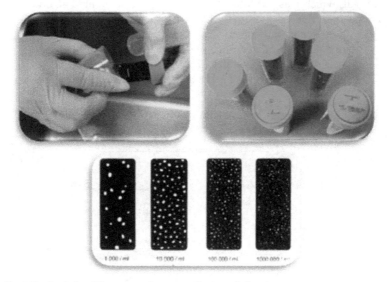

Fig. 10. Collect the lactobacillus sample, manufactured chart.

3.4 Plaque pH

Acidogenic bacteria in dental plaque metabolize carbohydrates rapidly getting acid as final product. The result is a change in pH of the plaque, as it relates to the time called the Stephan curve as a scheme to bring it takes a curve. The pH decreases rapidly in the first few minutes to gradually increase; it suggests that in 30 minutes should return to normal levels.

The caries activity test Cariostat®[4], developed by Shimono, is used to measure the decrease of pH caused by bacterial action in the plaque. It has been reported positive correlations between caries activity test score and the counts of SM and LB.

Not only can determine whether establishing new carious lesions, but also diagnose active or chronic lesions present (Nishimura et al., 1988; Lara-Carrillo et al., 2010b).

---

[4] Cariostat® (Dentsply-Sankin KK, Tokyo, Japan)

Munshi et al. (1999) reported a Cariostat® sensitivity of 96.7% and a specificity of 93.3%.

The procedure of Cariostat® is by changing color as a result of increased production of acids produced by fermentation of bacteria, is very sensitive and its relevance lies in its ability to predict the presence of caries in the future (Munshi et al., 1999).

It contains a high concentration of sucrose tryptose growth inhibitor of Gram-negative bacteria, with two types of indicators (green bromocresol and purple) to reveal visually the pH decrease in dental plaque (Ansai et al., 1994; Kornman, 2005; Nishimura et al., 1988a, 2008b).

A pH range of 4.0 ± 3 is considered high risk or marked caries activity.

Plaque is collected from buccal surfaces of first upper molars, using a sterilized cotton swab supplied in the kit, which was put into a test medium and incubated 48 hours at 37° C. The test color change is compared with the pattern provided by the manufacturer as follows:
Blue   negative value = pH 5.8-7.2
Green   one positive value = pH 5.4 ± 0.3
Yellow greenish   two positives value = pH 4.8 ± 0.3
Yellow   three positives value = pH < 4.4 (Fig. 11).

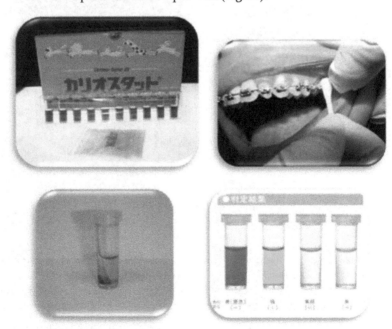

Fig. 11. Caries activity test Cariostat®.

3.5 Occult blood in saliva

The use of saliva for periodontal diagnosis has been subject to several investigations, which have been proposed for disease markers including proteins, cells, hormones, volatile components, ions, bacteria and bacterial products, among others.

It has become the leukocytes counts, in these salivary markers as an indicator of periodontal disease, since most of the salivary leukocytes entering to the oral cavity through the crevicular fluid when exist gingival inflammation, but these cells vary from person to person and even in one person can change during the day (Kaufman & Lamster, 2000).

Actually exists another colorimetric salivary test used as indicator at inflammation which involves determining occult blood derived from the gingival tissue for evaluates periodontal disease in initial stages, called Salivaster®[5] (Hashimoto et al., 2006; Niwa, & Fukuda, 1989).

The Salivaster® is a colorimetric test based on a catalytic reaction of hemoglobin in saliva inducing the formation of different colors ranging from yellow to dark green. The principle of the color reaction is similar to the test for blood in urine, but was developed for the particular viscosity of saliva (Fig. 12).

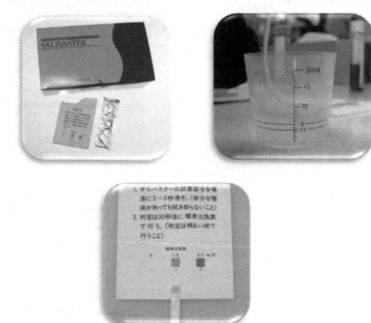

Fig. 12. Initial indicator of periodontal disease through occult blood in saliva (Salivaster®)

It is reported that this method has a sensitivity of 75.9% and a specificity of 90.5% for the detection of gingival inflammation (Kaufman & Lamster, 2000).

The procedure involves dipping the test paper in stimulated saliva for 2-3 seconds and then judging by comparing to the standard color change chart, divided into 3 levels:

Yellow   0.0 mg of blood per dL of saliva (no periodontal disease)
Llight blue   1.0 mg/dL (incipient periodontal disease)
Dark blue   2.5 mg/dL (periodontal disease present).

---

[5] Salivaster ® (Showa Yakuhin Kako Co. LTD, Tokyo, Japan)

3.6 Hygienic-dietary habits

This section covers those data on the frequency and quality of oral hygiene and consistency of diet, time and frequency of food intake.

There is little doubt that the change in lifestyle of civilization was resulting in an increase in the prevalence of dental caries, referring mainly to the increase of the diet of soft foods that contain carbohydrates.

Certain features of sugary foods and the conditions under which they are ingested, are more important in determining the cariogenic potential than amount of sugar (Moynihan, 2005).

The factors that establish the potential cariogenicity of sugary foods are:

- The physical consistency of the diet: food adhesives are more retentive than non-cariogenic.
- Time of ingestion: sugary foods are more dangerous when consumed between meals, as the natural defense mechanisms operate at maximum during meals. The worst time to cariogenic food is just before bedtime, because the mouth is dry by the circadian rhythm of saliva during sleep.
- The frequency: sugar intake reduces the pH of dental plaque that facilitates demineralization and promotes tooth decay, so that the more frequent the intake, more cariogenic foods become.

The severity of the above is that the sugars are rapidly degraded by bacteria in acidic metabolic end products, which will result in a greater demineralization process than remineralization with subsequent carious lesions.

But also, there are certain foods that can protect against the formation of dental caries by the substances that they contain in their structure, either because they are fibrous, fatty or protein, etc. which reduces their cariogenic potential, and when mixed with sugary foods, reduce the potential of the latter, these are called protective foods, among which we mention the cheese. It has been shown to finish a meal with cheese for dessert, reduces the acidity of the plaque and therefore tooth decay (cariostatic).

The cheese prevents enamel demineralization by two different mechanisms: by stimulating the flow of saliva, which buffers the plaque and by increasing concentrations of calcium and phosphorus in dental plaque, which promotes remineralization (Saroglu, 2007).

In recent years, has also increased the use of sweeteners and sugar substitutes; investigations have focused mainly on sugar alcohols (sorbitol, mannitol, maltitol and xylitol), starch hydrolysates (Lycasin), protein (Monellina) and synthetic chemicals (saccharin, cyclamate and aspartic). Unlike sugar, these are poorly metabolized by oral bacteria or metabolized by pathways that lead to acid formation. Even some of them reduce the bacterial metabolism and consequently the development of plaque on the oral tissues. Nutrition education is very important, also correct oral hygiene with effective brushing after every meal is basically in oral health, while considering preventive periodic revisions to the dentist.

The useful life of a toothbrush is determined more by the brushing method that the length of use. Its half-life is approximately three months; however, this estimate may vary due to differences in the brushing habits.

They have developed several methods of toothbrushing and most are identified by a single name like Bass, Stillman, Charters, or by a term indicating the main action to be taken: as spinning or massage.

The objectives of brushing are:

- Remove the plaque and stop the growth of it.
- Clean the teeth of food, debris and stains.
- Stimulate the gingival tissues.

Although the brush is the main mechanical means of plaque removal, often required of dental auxiliaries to remove residual plaque present in the proximal surfaces, among which include: dental floss, interdental cleaners, oral irrigators, mouth rinses buccal interdental sticks, and others (Klaus et al., 1991).

However, the majority of the population is disabled, unmotivated or are unaware of the need to devote time to remove the plaque from all tooth surfaces, or using products not suitable for removing plaque on the site crucial, or both.

To know the habits of the patient is recommended to apply a questionnaire which included a series of questions regarding daily brushing and eating habits, focusing on behavioral risk factors for dental disease. (Fig. 13).

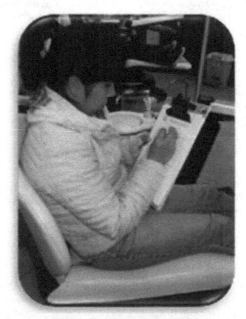

Fig. 13. Filling the questionnaire dietary and hygiene habits

4. Collection of samples

We recommended that patients brush their teeth three times a day using the Bass modified technique with toothpaste containing fluoride after placement of the appliances.

Recommendations to avoid retentive, cariogenic, or hard foods during orthodontic treatment were provided verbally.

For take the tests is necessary that the patients avoided eating or drinking and no toothbrushing at least 2 hours before taking the samples in both time points.

In our experience, with thirty-four subjects, where 14 males (mean age, 16.2 ± 3.4 years) and 20 females (mean age, 17.2 ± 6.3 years), we selected patients didn't have any systemic diseases, use of antibiotics at least 15 days before initiating the study, active caries, and on mixed dentition phase were excluded.

Two samples were taken from each patient, one before beginning the orthodontic treatment and the other 1 month after placement of the appliances, because this is the time for the appointment to change the first arch wire. The orthodontics attachments were placed in both arches.

Dental and skeletal diagnoses were obtained from each patient, defined by Angle's molar class and the subspinale-nasion-supramentale cephalometric angle (ANB). Fifteen patients had molar relation class I, fourteen had class II, four had class III, and in one patient it was not possible to determine the relationship due to absent first molars.

As for the skeletal diagnosis, fourteen were class I, nineteen were class II, and one were class III. The dental and skeletal diagnoses were not associated or determined the behavior of any of the studied variables (p>0.05) (data not shown).

4.1 Clinical markers

The mean DMFS index of the subjects was 6.47, although it was greater in females (8.70) that in males (3.28), these differences were not statistically significant (P = 0.1352. The mean O'Leary's plaque index was 44.6 %, males presented a slightly plaque percentage (50.84%) than females (40.15%; P = 0.1809) (data not shown).

4.2 Salivary markers

We did not find a statistically significant difference in the unstimulated salivary production before and 1-month after the placement of orthodontic appliances, nevertheless according to time point, in both samples, there were differences between the saliva production of males and females (P = 0.0026); specifically, the unstimulated salivary production was lower in women (Table 1).

The placement of orthodontic appliances promoted a major stimulated salivary flow in the subjects, with significant differences in the salivary production before and after treatment (P = 0.0001). The salivary stimulated flow rate was greater in males at the beginning (P = 0.0019; Table 1). The salivary buffer capacity showed differences after placement of the appliances (P = 0.0359) and between genders before the treatment (P = 0.0381) females showed lower capacity (Table 1).

Significant differences were observed in the salivary pH before and after treatment (P = 0.0246) with an increase of the pH value (Table 1).

Marker	Gender	Stages		Pa
		Before	After	
Salivary markers				
Unstimulated saliva (seconds)	Male	39.85 ± 19.17	38.64 ± 14.90	
	Female	45.65 ± 19.03	57.35 ± 17.43	0.4073
	pb	0.3903	0.0026*	
Stimulated saliva (mL/min)	Male	1.72 ± 0.65	1.76 ± 0.80	
	Female	1.06 ± 0.48	1.36 ± 0.50	0.0001*
	pb	0.0019*	0.0835	
Buffer capacity	Male	8.78 ± 2.19	8.71 ± 2.16	
	Female	6.90 ± 2.69	7.70 ± 1.59	0.0359*
	pb	0.0381*	0.1247	
Salivary pH	Male	7.68 ± 0.17	7.74 ± 0.09	
	Female	7.53 ± 0.38	7.73 ± 0.09	0.0246*
	pb	0.1672	0.7039	

Data shown as mean ± SD
pa value between before vs. after placement of appliances, based on paired t-test
pb value between genders, based on paired t-test
*P < 0.05

Table 1. Distribution of salivary markers by gender in the study (n = 34)

4.3 Bacterial markers

We observed changes in the CFU of SM after the placement of appliances. Before treatment 14/34 subjects had high values (>10^5); after one month of banding, 16/34 had high values.

In the first sample 7/34 subjects had high levels (>10^5) of LB, for the second sample we found 20/34 subjects in these same level, although statistically significant differences were not observed in the bacterial counts distribution (Table 2).

4.4 Plaque pH

The acidity of the initial plaque no registered significant modifications after the placement of appliances (P = 0.5467); however, we found differences between genders in the initial sample (P = 0.0430); the pH between 5.8-7.2 predominating in females, and lowest values (pH 5.4 ± 0.3) in males. The second sample showed more subjects with lowest values (pH 5.4 ± 0.3) in both genders (Table 2).

4.5 Occult blood in saliva

Differences were observed in the gingival bleeding before and after orthodontic treatment (P = 0.0305), with an increased the bleeding in saliva in the second sample. It has to be considered that in the beginning of the study most of the subjects were in the intermediate level with 1 mg/dL of occult blood in saliva (incipient periodontal disease) and one month later the periodontal disease present increase (Table 2).

| Marker | Stages | | | | P^a |
| | Before | | After | | |
	Male	Female	Male	Female	
Bacterial markers					
SM counts					
NC or $<10^3$	6	4	4	4	
$<10^5$	3	3	4	6	
$>10^5$ to 10^6	5	8	6	8	
$>10^6$	0	1	0	2	0.3741
P^b	0.8137		0.6416		
Lactobacillus counts					
NC	4	8	0	1	
10^3	3	5	4	4	
10^4	3	4	5	5	
10^5	2	3	8	8	
10^6	2	0	2	2	0.6905
P^b	0.4431		0.6832		
Plaque pH					
5.8 – 7.2	4	14	3	7	
5.4 ± 0.3	9	6	11	12	
4.8 ± 0.3	1	0	0	1	
< 4.4	0	0	0	0	0.5467
P^b	0.0430*		0.4414		
Occult blood in saliva					
No periodontal disease	1	1	0	0	
Incipient periodontal disease	8	15	8	15	
Periodontal disease present	5	4	6	5	0.0305*
	0.5432		0.2733		

NC = negative at culture
P^a value between before vs. after placement of appliances, based on X^2 test
P^b value between genders, based on X^2 test
* P < 0.05

Table 2. Distribution of bacterial markers, plaque pH and occult blood in saliva by gender in the study (n = 34)

It is established that orthodontic treatment induces changes in the oral environment, with increasing concentrations of mutans streptococci and lactobacilli, as well as increased blood concentration in saliva and decreased plaque pH.

This is exacerbated in stages which increase the use of attachments and the consequent difficulty of proper hygiene.

5. Conclusions

The clinical markers showed that males had lower DMFS index than females, nevertheless, the plaque index by O'Leary showed more plaque in males of this study.

The stimulated salivary flow increased after the placement of orthodontic appliances. In the present study it was greater in males, which is similar to international reports (Chang et al., 1999; Bretz et al., 2001; De Vigna et al., 2008).

The mean salivary flow rate for both genders was found in normal parameters: 1-3 mL/min in stimulated saliva and from 0.25-0.35 mL/min in unstimulated saliva. The variability of salivary flow rate has been established by other researchers (Torres et al, 2006).

The results support a direct and prolonged stimulatory effect after one month of treatment with fixed orthodontic appliances on salivary flow.

The saliva buffer capacity presented a significant increase in females after the orthodontic therapy. Males showed higher buffer capacity than females, this difference between genders have been demonstrated previously.

The salivary buffer capacity prevents the settling of pathogenic microorganisms in mouth, being an important risk indicator, because it reveals the response of the host.

Salivary pH demonstrated a significant increase in the 1st month of treatment, as opposed to other studies in which it has been demonstrated that the pH suffers alterations after 3 months of orthodontic treatment (Chang et al., 1999).

Males showed a more acid plaque pH at the beginning of the treatment, nevertheless an increase in acidity was demonstrated 1 month with orthodontic appliances in females. The plaque pH had significant differences between genders when the patients already were in orthodontic treatment.

The orthodontic appliances protected the plaque from the tooth brushing action, the mastication, and the salivary fluid. Accumulating more on the cervical region of the brackets or below the arches wire, which is the zone where a major demineralization can be found (Migale et al., 2009).

The present study showed an increase of CFU after placement of the orthodontic appliances, which has been demonstrated also by Chang (1999). Nevertheless, these changes in the 1st month of study were not statistically significant, as opposed to report by this same author.

Before initiating treatment, the majority of patients showed incipient periodontal disease detected trough the Salivaster® test, possibly caused by crowding, which in the majority of patients is the principal motivation for the orthodontic treatment. Likewise, a significant increase of periodontal disease was observed 1 month after initiating orthodontic therapy

(2.5 mg/dL of saliva). Inflammation of the adjacent connective tissue has been considered a consequence of the use of orthodontic bands, determining that the condition of the gum deteriorates during the treatment with fixed appliances, even in patients with good oral hygiene. (Lara-Carrillo et al., 2010a)

Checking the quality, pH and buffer capacity of saliva can be valuable as part of an overall clinical assessment, thus also monitoring bacterial counts, plaque and periodontal inflammation.

In conclusion, orthodontic treatment changes the oral environmental factors: promotes a major salivary stimulated flow and increases its buffer capacity and salivary pH, which increase the anticaries activity of saliva. Plaque pH did not demonstrate significant changes before and 1-month into orthodontic treatment. The bacterial levels did not increase significantly in the first month of the orthodontic treatment but, the increased of retentive surfaces rinsed the bleeding in saliva by periodontal injury.

Patients with orthodontic appliances require special care in terms of prevention caries and periodontal disease. For optimal patient care, it is necessary to analyzed if the changes during orthodontic treatment persist or change upon discontinuation of treatment.

The following markers emerged as protective factors: patients without active caries injuries increased significantly stimulated salivary flow, buffer capacity, and salivary pH, after placement orthodontic appliances.

In contrast, the following markers were negative risk factors to the oral environment: slightly increase in the infection levels of *SM* and *Lactobacillus*, and of occult blood in saliva.

Oral environment has the capacity of adjustment to the presence of a foreign body, increasing the salivary flow which contributes to the autoclisis and modifying the salivary composition to raise the pH and buffer capacity, it prevents colonization by potentially pathogenic microorganisms by denying them optimization of environmental conditions.

It is necessary to establish the parameters that the patient presents at the beginning and during the treatment, and determine which stages may show major changes, if these changes are kept or reversed during the course of the therapy, with the purpose of preventing in an opportune and effective way.

So it is advisable to develop a prevention protocol for the development of dental caries or enamel demineralization in patients at risk, as is the case of those who undergo orthodontic treatment with fixed appliances.

It is recognized that this type of treatment has the potential to cause damage to hard and soft tissues of the oral cavity. In patients undergoing orthodontic treatment with fixed appliances increases bacterial counts due to the favorable environment for the accumulation of plaque and food debris that increase the risk of tooth decay, coupled with the difficulty of plaque removal by conventional means of oral hygiene.

However, the best way to combat tooth decay and periodontal disease is the strict control of plaque, for which it has recommended the use of electric toothbrushes, mouthwashes, oral irrigators, and others. But one of the most important parts to maintain oral health is the motivation of the patient.

In this study it was observed that most patients showed interest in the results of their samples, from the very beginning knew the purpose of continually assessing their clinical characteristics, salivary and bacterial, asked if he had improved his health and brushing frequently controlled by plaque control record.

Because orthodontic appliances patients with an increased risk of tooth decay and/or periodontal disease problems, it is necessary to reduce the time in which these patients are at risk, the clinician will have the commitment of the good course of treatment, but the patient also plays an important role.

Another recommendation is to give greater publicity to the importance of oral health markers studied here can not only be applied in orthodontic patients, but in any patient is desirable to determine the risk of cavities that may have to take action convenient and proper preventive their clinical characteristics, salivary or bacterial infections, and especially those in which systemic disease is added.

6. References

Anderson P., Hector M.P. & Rampersad M.A. (2001). Critical pH in resting and stimulated whole saliva in groups of children and adults. *International Journal of Paediatric Dentistry*, Vol. 11, No.4 (July, 2001), pp. 266-273, ISSN 0960-7439.

Ansai T., Yamashita Y., Shibata Y., Katoh Y., Sakao S., Takamatsu N., Miyasaki H. & Takehara T. (1994). Relationship between dental caries experience of a group of Japanese kindergarten children and the results of two caries activity tests conducted on their saliva and dental plaque. *International Journal of Paediatric Dentistry*, Vol. 4, No.1 (March, 1994), pp. 13-17, ISSN 0960-7439.

Anusavice K.J. (2005). Present and future approaches for the control of caries. *Journal of Dental Education*, Vol. 69, No. 5 (May, 2005), pp. 538-554, ISSN 0022-0337.

Bollen A.M., Cunha-Cruz J., Bakko D.W., Huang G.J. & Hujoel P.P. (2008). The effects of orthodontic therapy on periodontal health. A systematic review of controlled evidence. *Journal of the American Dental Association*, Vol. 139, No. 4 (April 2008), pp 413-422, ISSN 0002-8177.

Bretz W.A., do Valle E.V., Jacobson J.J., Marchi F., Mendes S., Nor J.E., Cancado M.F. & Schneider L.G. (2001). Unstimulated salivary flow rates of young children. *Oral Surgery, Oral Medicine, Oral Pathology, Oral Radiology and Endodontics*, Vol 91, No. 5 (May 2001), pp 541-545, ISSN 1079-2104.

Butler B.L., Morejon O. & Low S.B. (1996). An accurate, time-efficient method to assess plaque accumulation. *Journal of the American Dental Association*, Vol. 127, No. 12 (December 1996), pp 1763-1766, ISSN 0002-8177.

Chang H.S., Walsh L.J. & Freer T.J. (1999). The effect of orthodontic treatment on salivary flow, pH, buffer capacity, and levels of mutans streptococci and lactobacilli. *Australian Orthodontic Journal*, Vol. 15, No. 4 (April 1999), pp 229-34, ISSN 0587-3908.

Dawes C. (2003). What is the critical pH and why does a tooth dissolve in acid? *Journal of the Canadian Dental Association*, Vol. 69, No. 11 (December 2003), pp 722-724, ISSN 0709-8936.

De Vigna A.P., Trindade G.A.M., Naval M.M.A., Soares L.A.A. & Reis A.L. (2008). Saliva composition and functions: A comprehensive review. *The Journal of Contemporary Dental Practice*, Vol. 9, No. 3 (March 2008), pp 72-80, ISSN 1526-3711.

Derks A., Kuijpers-Jagtman A.M., Frencken J.E., Van't Hof M. & Katsaros Ch. (2007). Caries preventive measures used in orthodontic practices: An evidence-based decision? *American Journal of Orthodontics and Dentofacial Orthopedics*, Vol. 132, No. 2 (August 2007), pp 165-170, ISNN 0889-5406.

Featherstone J. (2000). The science and practice of caries prevention. *Journal of the American Dental Association*, Vol. 131, No. 7 (July 2000), pp 887-899, ISSN 0002-8177.

Fenoll-Palomares C., Muñoz-Montagud J.V., Sanchiz V., Herreros B., Hernández V., Mínguez M. & Benages A. (2004). Unstimulated salivary flow rate, pH and buffer capacity of saliva in healthy volunteers. *Revista Española de Enfermedades Digestivas*, Vol. 96, No. 11 (November 2004), pp 773-783, ISSN 1130-0108.

Gwinnett A.J. & Ceen R.F. (1979). Plaque distribution on bonded brackets: a scanning microscope study. *American Journal of Orthodontics and Oral Surgery*, Vol. 75, No. 6 (June 1979), pp 667-677, ISSN 0002-9416.

Harris N. & García-Godoy F. (2001). *Preventive primary dentistry* (2nd edition), Editorial El Manual Moderno, ISBN 0-83857898-5, México. [In Spanish].

Hashimoto M., Yamanaka K., Shimosato T., Ozawa A., Takigawa T., Hidaka S., Sakai T & Noguchi T. (2006). Oral condition and health status of elderly 8020 achievers in Aichi Prefecture. *The Bulletin of Tokyo Dental College*, No. 47, vol. 2 (May 2006), pp 37-43, ISSN 0040-8891.

Heintze S.D., Finke C, Jost-Brinkman P-G & Miethke R.R. (1999). *Oral Health for the Orthodontic patient*. Quintessence Publishing Co., ISBN 0-86715-295-8, Hong Kong.

Jensen B., Bratthall D. (1989). A new method for the estimation of Mutans Streptococci in human saliva. *Journal of Dental Research*, Vol. 68, No. 3 (March 1989), pp 468-471, ISSN 0022-0345.

Katz S, Mc Donald J.L., Stookey G.K. (1997). *Preventive dentistry in action*. Editorial Panamericana, ISBN 968-7157-08-9, México. [In Spanish].

Kaufman E. & Lamster I. (2000). Analysis of saliva for periodontal diagnosis- a review. *Journal of Clinical Periodontology*, Vol. 27, No. 7 (July 2000), pp 453-465, ISSN 0303-6979.

Klaus H., Rateitschak E.M & Wolf H.F. (1991). Pedodontics Atlas (2nd edition), Salvat, ISBN 84-345-2535-6, Barcelona. [In Spanish].

Kornman K.S. (2005). Diagnostic and prognostic tests for oral disease: practical applications. *Journal of Dental Education*, Vol. 69, No. 5 (May, 2005), pp. 498-508, ISSN 0022-0337.

Lara-Carrillo E., Montiel-Bastida N.M., Sánchez-Pérez L., Alanís-Tavira J.(2010). Changes in the oral environment during four stages of orthodontic treatment. *Korean Journal of Orthodontics*, Vol. 40, No. 2 (April 2010), pp 95-105, ISSN 1225-5610.

Lara-Carrillo E., Montiel-Bastida N.M., Sánchez-Pérez L., Alanís-Tavira J. (2010). Effect of orthodontic treatment on saliva, plaque and the levels of Streptococcus mutans and Lactobacillus. *Medicina Oral Patología Oral y Cirugía Bucal*, Vol. 15, No. 6 (November 2010), pp 924-9, ISSN 1698-4447.

Larmas M. (1992). Saliva and dental caries: diagnostic tests for normal dental practice. *International Dental Journal*, Vol. 42, No. 4 (August 1992), pp 199-208, ISSN 0020-6539.

Leone C.W. & Oppenheim F.G. (2001). Physical and chemical aspects of saliva as indicators of risk for dental caries in humans. *Journal of Dental Education*, Vol. 65, No. 10 (October, 2001), pp. 1054-1061, ISSN 0022-0337.

Menaker L., Mohart R.E. & Navia J.M. (1986). *Biological basis of dental caries*, Salvat, ISBN 84-345-2142-3, Barcelona. [In Spanish].

Migale D., Barbato E., Bossú M., Ferro R., Ottolenght L. (2009). Oral health and malocclusion in 10 to 11 years-old children in southern Italy. *European Journal of Paediatric Dentistry*, Vol. 10, No. 1 (March 2009), pp 13-18, ISSN 1591-996X.

Monterde C.M.E., Delgado R.J.M., Martínez R.I.M., Guzmán F.C.E., Espejel M.M. (2002). Demineralization-remineralization in the dental enamel. *Revista ADM*, Vol. 59, No. 6 (November-December 2002), pp 220-222, ISSN 0001-0944. [In Spanish].

Moynihan P. J. (2005). The role of diet and nutrition in the etiology and prevention of oral diseases. *Bulletin of the World Health Organization*, Vol. 83, No. 9 (September 2005), pp 694-699, ISSN 0042-9686.

Munshi A.K., Hedge A.M. & Munshi A. (1999). Relationship between the existing caries status, plaque, S. mutans and Cariostat caries activity test in children. *Journal of Indian Society of Pedodontics and Preventive Dentistry*, Vol. 17, No. 3 (September 1999), pp 73-89, ISSN 0970-4388.

National Institutes of Health Consensus Development conference statement. (2001). Diagnosis and management of dental caries throughout life, march 26-28. *Journal of the American Dental Association*, Vol. 132, No. 8 (August 2001), pp 1153-1161, ISSN 0002-8177.

Nishimura M., Bhuiyan M.M., Matsumura S & Shimono T. (1988). Assessment of the caries activity test (Cariostat) based on the infection levels of mutans streptococci and lactobacillos in 2 to 13 year old children's dental plaque. *ASDC Journal of Dentistry for Children*, Vol. 65, No. 4 (July-August 1988), pp 248-251, ISSN 1945-1954.

Nishimura M., Oda T., Kariya N., Matsumura S. & Shimono T. (2008). Using a caries activity test to predict caries risk in early childhood. *Journal of the American Dental Association*, Vol. 139, No. 1 (January 2008), pp 63-71, ISSN 0002-8177.

Niwa M. & Fukuda M. (1989). Clinical study on the control of dental plaque using a photo energy conversion a toothbrush equipped with a TiO_2 semiconductor. *Shigaku*, Vol. 77, No. 2 (August 1989), pp 1-16, ISSN 0029-8484.

O' Leary T.J., Drake R.B. & Naylor J.E. (1972). The plaque control record. *Journal of Periodontology*, Vol. 43, No. 1 (January 1972), pp 38, ISSN 0022-3492.

Prieto V.J.M. & Yuste J.R. (2010). *Balcells. The clinic and the laboratory. Interpretation of analysis and functional tests* (21st edition), Elsevier Masson, ISBN 9-78844-582030-8, España. [In Spanish].

Proffit W.R. (2008). *Contemporary Orthodontics*. (4th. Edition), Elsevier Mosby, ISBN 978-84-8086-330-8, España. [In Spanish].

Sánchez P.L. & Sáenz M.L.P. (2003). A comparison between risk caries indicators. *Boletin Médico del Hospital Infantil de México*. No. 60, Vol. 3, (May-June 2003), pp 263-273, ISSN 1665-1146. [In Spanish]

Sánchez P.T.L. & Sáenz M.L.P. (1998). Caries experience as predictors of disease at 18 months. *Revista ADM*, Vol. 55, No. 6 (November-December 1998), pp 283-286, ISSN 0001-0944. [In Spanish].

Saroglu S. & Aras S. (2007). Effect of white cheese and sugarless yoghurt on dental plaque acidogenicity. *Caries Research*, Vol. 41 No. 3 (March 2007), pp 208-211, ISSN 0008-6568.

Sidlauskas A. & Lopatiené K. (2009). The prevalence of malocclusion among 7-15 years-old Lithuanian schoolchildren. *Medicina (Kaunas), Vol.* 45 No. 2 (February 2009), pp 147-152, ISSN 1010-660X.

Tanzer J.M., Livingston J. & Thompson A. (2001). The microbiology of primary dental caries in humans. *Journal of Dental Education*, Vol. 65, No. 10 (October, 2001), pp. 1028-1037, ISSN 0022-0337.

Torres S.R., Nucci M., Milanos E., Pessoa P.R., Massaud A. & Munhoz T. (2006). Variations of salivary flow rates in Brazilian school children. *Brazilian Oral Research*, Vol. 20 No. 1 (January-March 2006), pp 8-12, ISSN 1806-8324.

Trulsson U., Strandmark M., Mohlin B. & Berggren U. (2002). A qualitative study of teenagers' decision to undergo orthodontic treatment with fixed appliance. *Journal of Orthodontics*, Vol. 29, No. 3 (September 2002), pp 197-204, ISSN 1465-3125.

Turbill E.A., Richmond S. & Wright J.L. (2001). The time-factor in orthodontics: What influences the duration of treatments in National Health Service practices? *Community Dentistry and Oral Epidemiology*, Vol. 29 No. 1 (February 2001), pp 62-72, ISSN 0301-5661.

Varma S., Banerjee A. & Bartlett D. (2008). An in vivo investigation of associations between saliva properties, caries prevalence and potential lesion activity in an adult UK population. *Journal of Dentistry*, Vol. 36 No. 4 (April 2008), pp 294-299, ISSN 0300-5712.

WHO Oral Health Country/Area Profile Programme. (July 17, 2011). Caries prevalence: DMFT and DMFS. August 23, 2011, Available from:
    http://www.mah.se/CAPP/Methods-and-Indices/for-Caries-prevalence/

WHO Oral Health Country/Area Profile Programme. (July 5, 2011). The plaque control record (O'Leary T, Drake R, Taylor, 1972). August 23, 2011, Available from:
    http://www.mah.se/CAPP/Methods-and-Indices/Oral-Hygiene-Indices/Plaque-Control-Record/

World Health Organization. (1997). *Oral Health Surveys. Basic methods.* (4th edition), W.H.O, ISNB 9-78924-154493-1, Geneva.

Zárate D.A.S., Leyva H.E.R. & Franco M.F. (2004). Determination of pH and total proteins in saliva in patients with and without fixed orthodontic appliances (pilot study). *Revista Odontológica Mexicana*, Vol. 8 No. 3 (September 2004), pp 59-63 ISSN 1870-199X. [In Spanish].

9

The Dental Volumetric Tomography, RVG, and Conventional Radiography in Determination the Depth of Approximal Caries

Cafer Türkmen, Gökhan Yamaner and Bülent Topbaşı
Department of Operative Dentistry,
Faculty of Dentistry, University of Marmara, Istanbul,
Turkey

1. Introduction

Detection of carious lesions is prerequisite to an optimal preventive and minimal surgical intervention strategy. Radiographs are the most accurate diagnostic aid available for the detection of alveolar osseous abnormalities and dental disease progression (Russel & Pitts, 1993; Rothman, 1998). The development of digital radiography (radiovisiographs-RVG) has created new options in dentistry (Hedrick et al., 1994; Svanæs et al., 2000; Van der Stelt, 2005). However, imaging systems used in dentistry are largely limited to 2 dimensional (2-D) systems in including conventional-based radiography and digital radiography. The problem inherent to 2-D system is that 3 dimensional anatomy is collapsed into 2-D space, resulting in the superimposition of structures that potentially obscure features of interest and decrease diagnostic sensitivity. There are a number of 3-D systems available, like computed tomography (CT), tuned aperture computed tomography (TACT), and cone beam computed tomography (CBCT) (Hedrick et al., 1998; Mozzo et al., 1998; Sukovic, 2003; Aranyarachkul et al., 2005; Walker et al., 2005).

The CBCT technique presents an innovation of tomographic imaging systems and subsequent volumetric image reconstruction for dentistry. When compared with other methods of tomographic imaging, CBCT is characterized by rapid volumetric image acquisition from a single low radiation dose scan of the patient. CBCT, also known as true volumetric computed tomography (TVCT) designed for use in dental imaging of osseous structures has been introduced (Rothman, 1998; Mozzo et al., 1998; Schulze et al., 2005). The first available and now well-established CBCT system, the NewTom is an example of such a CBCT machine dedicated to dental and maxillofacial imaging, particularly for surgical and/or prosthetics implant planning in the field of dentistry. The NewTom differs from a traditional dental CT scan in the way it captures an image; it does so by cone beam volumetric tomography. The W-ray tube revolves around the patient's head in a single spiral, capturing a volume with each of the 360 degrees it rotates. Added together, the volumetric cone images are reformatted without any discernible error. In fact, the NewTom is accurate to 0.1 mm. While a dental CT scan takes ten minutes of working time and exposes the patient to two minutes of radiation, the NewTom scan takes 70 seconds and exposes the patient to 17 seconds of low-dose radiation. The radiation from a NewTom scan is comparable to the radiation from a single Panorex, while a dental CT scan is roughly equivalent to 6-8 times that amount, depending on bone density.

It is also possible to detect the relationship of the caries lesions with pulp chamber as 3-D. Therefore, the superpositions were eliminated with this system. The aim of this study was to compare the new dental volumetric tomography, RVG and conventional radiography in determination of the depth of approximal carious lesions.

2. Materials & methods

Randomly chosen 44 extracted and unrestored premolars and molars teeth with appoximal carious lesions were embedded in silicone (Optosil- Bayer Dental, Leverkusen, FRG) blocks in sets of 4 (2 premolars and 2 molars in contact), simulating as far as possible their presumed anatomical relationships. Extra 3 posterior teeth (One of them with a 1 cm metal wire fixed on occlusal, the others drilled in depth of 3 mm round hole in proximal contacts) were mounted for the calibration and control.

D (Agfa Dentus M 2D, Germany) and E (Cea Dent, Ced D, Sweden) – speed radiographic films were used to take x-ray. Exposures were standardized at 18 impulses (0.3 s) from a model Kodak C6 320 FFD (70 kVp, 8 mA) radiation source (Kodak-Trophy ETX, France) that is also then integrated with the imaging system *(Kodak RVG 5000)* with distance of 20 cm holder device (short cone) (Dentsply Gendex Rinn, Milano, Italy). Films were processed immediately after exposure in fresh Kodak Readymatic processing solutions by means of a Velopex automatic temperature controlled processor (Extra-x, London, England). Processed radiographs were scanned to the computer for the measurement of carious lesions depths linearly in software. For the digital imaging, the sensor was fixed with the holder and Trophy dental unit was exposed for the 0.18 s.

The NewTom (NewTom 9000; Quantitative Radiology, Verona, Italy) CBCT machine was used for the volumetric CT imaging. The teeth blocks were inserted to the centre of a water filled glass model have a volume to simulate a human head. Exposure was; 110 kVp, 5,2 mA for 36 s.

The depth of carious lesions was measured linearly in software (NewTom 3G, generation 2).

For the validation criteria, the roots of teeth were discarded and the crowns were sectioned as mesiodistally by a low speed diamond saw (Isomet 100 precission saw, Buchler, Germany) for histological measurements under the stereomicropcopy (Leica MZ 75, Heerbrugg, Germany).

Bland-Altman plot test was used to describe agreement between software and histologic measurements of approximal carious lesion depths.

3. Results

Table 1 lists the measured the average carious lesion depths of 44 teeth on digital images (radiograps, RVG, and tomographic) and histologic observation.

The Bland-Altman plot test revealed that the percentage agreement between radiographic and histologic measurements was 93.2% while 6.8% of the points were beyond the ±2 (Std. Dev.) of the mean difference. On the other hand, 90.9% agreement were observed between both RVG and histologic measurement and volumetric CT and histologic measurement. 9.1% of the points were beyond the ±2 (SD) of the mean difference for both comparisons.

Tooth No	Radiographic	RVG	Volumetric CT	Histologic
1	2.3	2.5	2.6	2.4
2	3.3	3.3	3.5	3.2
3	4.8	4.9	5.0	4.7
4	4.4	4.5	4.7	4.3
5	2.6	2.6	2.5	2.3
6	3.0	3.1	3.3	3.0
7	4.4	4.5	4.4	4.2
8	4.8	4.9	5.1	4.7
9	3.5	3.5	3.6	3.3
10	2.0	2.1	2.2	2.0
11	4.1	4.0	4.2	3.8
12	4.3	4.4	4.6	4.2
13	3.2	3.1	3.3	3.0
14	3.0	3.1	3.2	2.8
15	4.0	4.1	4.1	3.8
16	3.6	3.7	3.8	3.5
17	3.8	3.8	3.9	3.6
18	4.3	4.2	4.4	4.1
19	4.7	4.8	4.7	4.2
20	4.6	4.8	4.9	4.6
21	2.3	2.4	2.6	2.3
22	2.5	2.5	2.7	2.4
23	2.7	2.9	2.9	2.8
24	3.6	3.8	3.7	3.5
25	4.4	4.6	4.8	4.1
26	3.6	3.7	3.9	3.8
27	2.1	2.3	2.3	2.0
28	4.3	4.0	4.4	4.1
29	3.0	3.3	3.5	3.2
30	2.7	2.9	3.0	2.5
31	3.1	3.2	3.4	3.0
32	4.0	4.1	4.3	3.8
33	3.5	3.5	3.7	3.3
34	2.6	2.7	2.7	2.7
35	2.8	2.6	2.9	2.5
36	4.2	4.3	4.4	4.0
37	3.3	3.4	3.6	3.2
38	3.5	3.7	3.9	3.4
39	4.0	4.2	4.4	3.9
40	3.8	3.3	3.5	4.0
41	2.7	2.6	2.7	4.1
42	1.8	2.0	2.1	4.2
43	1.4	1.7	1.5	4.3
44	2.3	2.3	2.5	4.4

(Bland-Altman analysis: Radiographic-histologic: 93.2%, RVG-histologic and Volumetric-histologic: 90.9%)

Table 1. Carious lesion depths (mm) measured linearly in software and histologically.

The stereomicroscopy measurements revealed that the real caries depth was determined with the new volumetric tomography (fig.1) while RVG (fig.2) and similarly conventional radiography (fig.3) imaged less depth than it.

Histologic examination of the teeth confirmed that the dental volumetric CT also appears to be very promising in caries lesion imaging.

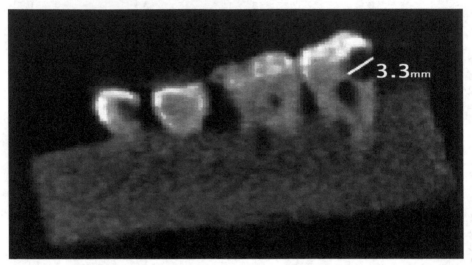

Fig. 1. Digital image of Volumetric CT.

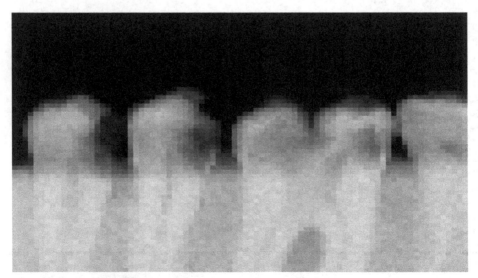

Fig. 2. Digital image of RVG.

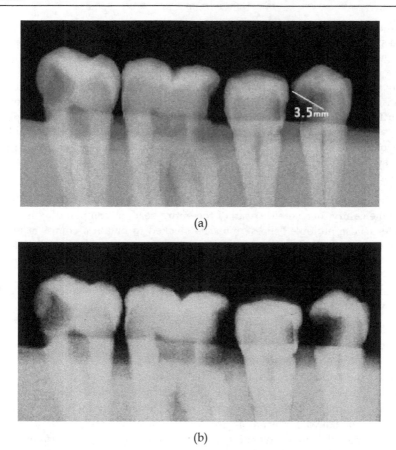

(a)

(b)

Fig. 3. Photographs of conventional radiographs, D (a) and E (b) speed films.

4. Discussion

The present study has demonstrated that the volumetric tomography images have the
potential to be the practical extraoral imaging modality for proximal caries detection.

In the most of studies (Velders et al., 1996; Svanæs et al., 2000; Wenzel, 2001; Khan et al.,
2004; Young & Featherstone, 2005), the proximal carious lesion was evaluated by using the
visual criterion. Although the visual criterion used was somewhat subjective, it represented
the best clinical representation of a proximal carious lesion. In previous similar in vitro
studies (Jesse, 1999; Kooistra et al., 2005), the gold standard for comparisons was histological
section of the extracted teeth. Caries depth was evaluated in these sections based solely on
the microscopic evaluation of a color change between involved and uninvolved dentin.

The singular purpose of the radiographic capture device (DDR sensor or conventional film)
is to capture the X-ray photon density pattern as it emerges from the subject tissues. The
photon dispersion pattern that emerges from the tissues is a function of the tissues and the
radiation source. An image would be sharper if the beam originated from a point source

rather than a source area. Clinical radiation generators emit X-rays from a source area and not from a singular point. This means that radiographic images are subject to loss of image detail and geometric unsharpness. The loss of image detail and sharpness is a function of the dimensions of the focal spot. The greater the focal spot size, the greater the loss of detail. Since X-ray photons cannot be focused into a sharp image as light can be focused through a camera lens, the image captured by conventional film or DDR sensors will never have a crisp, in focus appearance like a photograph focused through a lens. Radiographic images will always be subject to a certain degree of geometric unsharpness that will limit the resolution of the image that can be captured. The photon dispersion pattern cannot be improved by the sensor and will continue to limit image quality and sharpness for both conventional and DDR systems (Langland & Sippy, 1973; Hedrick et al., 1994).

The CBCT scanners utilize a two-dimensional, or panel, detector, which allows for a single rotation of the gantry to generate a scan of the entire head, as compared with conventional CT scanners whose multiple "slices" must be stacked to obtain a complete image. Cone beam technology utilizes X-rays much more efficiently, requires far less electrical energy, and allows for the use of smaller and less expensive X-ray components than fan-beam technology. In addition, the fan-beam technology used in conventional CT scanners does not lend itself to miniaturization because it requires significant space to spiral around the entire body (Sukovic, 2003; Marmulla et al., 2005).

Jaffray & Siewerdsen (2000) noted that the CBCT approach offers two important features that dramatically reduce its cost in comparison to a conventional scanner. First, the cone beam nature of the acquisition does not require an additional mechanism to move the patient during the acquisition. Second, the use of a cone beam, as opposed to a fan beam, significantly increases the X-ray utilization, lowering the X-ray tube heat capacity required for volumetric scanning. For the same source and detector geometry, the efficiency roughly scales with slice thickness. For example, the X-ray utilization increases by a factor of 30 in going from a 3 mm slice in a conventional scanner to a cone angle corresponding to a 100 mm slice with a cone beam system. This would reduce heat load capacity dramatically.

In summary, cone beam CT is a versatile emerging technology whose high and isotropic spatial resolution, undistorted images, compact size and relatively low cost, make it a perfect candidate for a dedicated dentomaxillofacial imaging modality. When combined with dedicated software packages, it can provide practitioners with a complete solution for demanding tasks (Mozzo et al., 1998; Sukovic, 2003; Schulze et al., 2005).

For approximal caries detection, the sensitivity of the volumetric dental tomography images was found to be slightly less than conventional radiographs and digital images in this study. Overall, the three methods were not statistically significantly different for the determination depth of the approximal carious lesions in vitro.

5. Conclusion

The results from the initial study suggest that although the sensitivities determined for all techniques were low, the volumetric dental tomography images showed that this device had a potential for detection approximal caries depths, root canal filling lengths, and left emptiness in the root in 3-D views.

6. References

Aranyarachkul, P.; Caruso, J., Gantes, B., Riggs, M., Dus, I. & Yamada, J. M. (2005). Bone density assessments of dental implant sites: 2. quantitative cone-beam computerized tomography. *International Journal of Oral & Maxillofacial Implants*, Vol. 20, pp. 416-424.

Hedrick, R.T.; Dove, B., Peters, D.D. & McDavid, W.D. (1994). Radiographic determination of canal length: Direct digital radiography versus conventional radiography. *Journal of Endodontics*, Vol. 20, pp. 320-326.

Jaffray, D.A. & Siewerdsen, J.H. (2000). Cone-beam computed tomography with a flat-panel imager: Initial performance characterization. *Medical Physics*, Vol. 27, pp. 1311-1323.

Jesse, S.A.; Makins, S.R. & Bretz, W.A. (1999). Accuracy of proximal caries depth determination using two intraoral film speeds. *General Dentistry*, Vol. 47, pp. 88-93.

Khan, E.A.; Tyndall, D.A. & Caplan, D. (2004). Extraoral imaging for proximal caries detection: Bitewings vs scanogram. *Oral Surgery Oral Medicine Oral Pathology Oral Radiology & Endodontics*, Vol. 98, pp. 730-737.

Kooistra, S.; Dennison, J.B., Yaman, P., Burt, B.A. & Taylor, G.W. (2005). Radiographic versus clinical extension of class II carious lesions using an F-speed film. *Operative Dentistry*, Vol. 30, pp. 719-726.

Langland, O.E. & Sippy, F.H. (2005). Textbook of dental radiography. 1st edn. Springfield: Charles C Thomas, 1973.

Marmulla, R.; Wörtche, R., Mühling, J. & Hassfeld, S. (2005). Geometric accuracy of the NewTom 9000 Cone Beam CT. *Dentomaxillofacial Radiology*, Vol. 34, pp. 28-31.

Mozzo, P.; Procacci, C., Tacconi, A., Tinazzi Martini, P. & Bergamo Andtreis, I.A. (1998). A new volumetric CT machine for dental imaging based on the cone-beam technique: preliminary results. *European Radiology*, Vol. 8, pp. 1558-1564.

Rothman, S.L.G. (1998). *Dental applications of computerized tomography*. 1st Edn. Quintessence Publishing Co, Inc., Illionis, pp. 5-57.

Russell, M. & Pitts, N.B. (1993). Radiovisiographic diagnosis of dental caries: Initial comparison of basic mode videoprints with bitewing radiography. *Caries Research*, Vol. 27, pp. 65-70.

Schulze, D.; Heiland, M., Blake, F., Rother, U. & Schmelzle, R. (2005). Evaluation of quality of reformatted images from two cone-beam computed tomographic systems. *Journal of Cranio-Maxillofacial Surgery*, Vol. 33, pp. 19-23.

Sukovic, P. (2003). Cone beam computed tomography in craniofacial imaging. *Orthodontics of Craniofacial Restorations*, Vol. 6, pp. 31-36.

Svanæs, D.B.; Møystad, A. & Larheim, T.A. (2000). Approximal caries depth assessment with storage phosphor versus film radiography. *Caries Research*, Vol.34, pp. 448-453.

Van der Stelt, P.F. (2005). Filmless imaging: The uses of digital radiography in dental practice. *Journal of American Dental Association*, Vol. 136, pp. 1379-1387.

Velders, X.L.; Sanderink, G.C.H. & Van der Stelt, P.F. (1996). Dose reduction of two digital sensor systems measuring file lengths. *Oral Surgery, Oral Medicine Oral Pathology Oral Radiology & Endodontics*, Vol. 81, pp. 607-612.

Walker, L.; Enciso, R. & Mah, J. (2005). Three-dimensional localization of maxillary canines with cone-beam computed tomography. *American Journal of Orthodontic & Dentofacial Orthopedics*, Vol. 128, pp. 418-423.

Wenzel, A. (2001). Computer-automated caries detection in digital bitewings: Consistency of a program and its influence on observer agreement. *Caries Research*, Vol. 35, pp. 12-20.

Young, D.A. & Featherstone, J.D.B. (2005). Digital imaging fiber-optic trans-illumination, F-speed radiographic film and depth of approximal lesions. *Journal of American Dental Association*, Vol. 136, pp. 1682-1687.

Permissions

The contributors of this book come from diverse backgrounds, making this book a truly international effort. This book will bring forth new frontiers with its revolutionizing research information and detailed analysis of the nascent developments around the world.

We would like to thank LI, Ming-yu, for lending his expertise to make the book truly unique. He has played a crucial role in the development of this book. Without his invaluable contribution this book wouldn't have been possible. He has made vital efforts to compile up to date information on the varied aspects of this subject to make this book a valuable addition to the collection of many professionals and students.

This book was conceptualized with the vision of imparting up-to-date information and advanced data in this field. To ensure the same, a matchless editorial board was set up. Every individual on the board went through rigorous rounds of assessment to prove their worth. After which they invested a large part of their time researching and compiling the most relevant data for our readers. Conferences and sessions were held from time to time between the editorial board and the contributing authors to present the data in the most comprehensible form. The editorial team has worked tirelessly to provide valuable and valid information to help people across the globe.

Every chapter published in this book has been scrutinized by our experts. Their significance has been extensively debated. The topics covered herein carry significant findings which will fuel the growth of the discipline. They may even be implemented as practical applications or may be referred to as a beginning point for another development. Chapters in this book were first published by InTech; hereby published with permission under the Creative Commons Attribution License or equivalent.

The editorial board has been involved in producing this book since its inception. They have spent rigorous hours researching and exploring the diverse topics which have resulted in the successful publishing of this book. They have passed on their knowledge of decades through this book. To expedite this challenging task, the publisher supported the team at every step. A small team of assistant editors was also appointed to further simplify the editing procedure and attain best results for the readers.

Our editorial team has been hand-picked from every corner of the world. Their multi-ethnicity adds dynamic inputs to the discussions which result in innovative outcomes. These outcomes are then further discussed with the researchers and contributors who give their valuable feedback and opinion regarding the same. The feedback is then collaborated with the researches and they are edited in a comprehensive manner to aid the understanding of the subject.

Apart from the editorial board, the designing team has also invested a significant amount of their time in understanding the subject and creating the most relevant covers. They scrutinized every image to scout for the most suitable representation of the subject and create an appropriate cover for the book.

The publishing team has been involved in this book since its early stages. They were actively engaged in every process, be it collecting the data, connecting with the contributors or procuring relevant information. The team has been an ardent support to the editorial, designing and production team. Their endless efforts to recruit the best for this project, has resulted in the accomplishment of this book. They are a veteran in the field of academics and their pool of knowledge is as vast as their experience in printing. Their expertise and guidance has proved useful at every step. Their uncompromising quality standards have made this book an exceptional effort. Their encouragement from time to time has been an inspiration for everyone.

The publisher and the editorial board hope that this book will prove to be a valuable piece of knowledge for researchers, students, practitioners and scholars across the globe.

List of Contributors

Luis Pezo Lanfranco and Sabine Eggers
Laboratório de Antropologia Biológica, Depto. de Genética e Biologia Evolutiva, Instituto de Biociências, Universidade de São Paulo, Brazil

Amila Brkić
Sarajevo University, School of Dental Medicine, Department of Oral Surgery and Dental Implantology, Sarajevo, Bosnia and Herzegovina

Virginie Gonzalez-Garcin1 and Gaëlle Soulard
UMR 5199 PACEA, Anthropologie des Populations Passées et Présentes, Université Bordeaux1, Talence, France

Petr Velemínský
Department of Anthropology, National Museum, Prague, Czech Republic

Petra Stránská
Institute of Archaeology, Academy of Sciences of the Czech Republic, Prague, Czech Republic

Jaroslav Bruzek
UMR 5199 PACEA, Anthropologie des Populations Passées et Présentes, Université Bordeaux1, Talence, France
Department of Anthropology, Faculty of Humanities, West Bohemian University, Pilsen, Czech Republic

Hüseyin Tezel and Hande Kemaloğlu
Ege University, Faculty of Dentistry, Department of Restorative Dentistry and Endodontics, Izmir, Turkey

David Todem
Division of Biostatistics, Department of Epidemiology and Biostatistics, Michigan State University, East Lansing, MI, USA

Camilo Abalos, Amparo Jiménez-Planas,
Elena Guerrero, Manuela Herrera and Rafael Llamas, University of Seville, School Dentistry, Spain

Michele Baffi Diniz1
Cruzeiro do Sul University, Brazil

Jonas de Almeida Rodrigues
Federal University of Rio Grande do Sul, Brazil

Adrian Lussi
University of Bern, Switzerland

Edith Lara-Carrillo
Faculty of Dentistry, Autonomous University of the State of Mexico, Mexico

Cafer Türkmen, Gökhan Yamaner and Bülent Topbaşı
Department of Operative Dentistry, Faculty of Dentistry, University of Marmara, Istanbul, Turkey

Printed in the USA
CPSIA information can be obtained
at www.ICGtesting.com
JSHW011359221024
72173JS00003B/341

9 781632 423603